# A Place to Call Home

## Long-Term Care in Canada

Edited by Pat Armstrong, Madeline Boscoe, Barbara Clow,
Karen Grant, Margaret Haworth-Brockman, Beth Jackson,
Ann Pederson, Morgan Seeley and Jane Springer

Fernwood Publishing • Halifax & Winnipeg

Editing: Jane Springer
Cover design: John van der Woude
Printed and bound in Canada by Hignell Book Printing
Printed on paper containing 100% post-consumer fibre.

Published in Canada by Fernwood Publishing
32 Oceanvista Lane
Black Point, Nova Scotia, B0J 1B0
and #8 - 222 Osborne Street, Winnipeg, Manitoba, R3L 1Z3
www.fernwoodpublishing.ca


Fernwood Publishing Company Limited gratefully acknowledges the financial support
of the Government of Canada through the Book Publishing Industry Development
Program (BPIDP), the Canada Council for the Arts and the Nova Scotia
Department of Tourism and Culture for our publishing program.

Library and Archives Canada Cataloguing in Publication

A place to call home: long-term care in Canada / Pat Armstrong ... [et al.].

ISBN 978-1-55266-293-9

1. Long-term care of the sick--Canada. 2. Long-term care facilities--Canada.
I. Armstrong, Pat, 1945-

RA998.C3P53 2009      362.160971      C2008-907798-9

# Contents

# Acknowledgements

This book was made possible by all those who participated in the workshop "Designing Long-Term Residential Care with Women in Mind." Brought together by Women and Health Care Reform — working in cooperation with the Atlantic Centre of Excellence for Women's Health — researchers, policy-makers and practitioners collaborated to develop gender-sensitive ideas and practices that could lead to promising conditions for workers and residents in long-term care. Their energy and commitment were critical to the development of this book and we thank them for taking the time to care. Women and Health Care Reform receives financial support from the Women's Health Contribution Program of the Bureau of Women's Health and Gender Analysis at Health Canada. The views expressed here do not necessarily represent the views of Health Canada.

# Contributors

PAT ARMSTRONG is a professor of Sociology and Women's Studies at York University and holds a Canadian Health Services Research Foundation and Canadian Institutes of Health Research Chair. She is co-author or editor of numerous books, peer-reviewed articles and technical reports on women's health-related issues, women's work and social policy. Her books include *Women's Health, Critical to Care* and *About Canada*.

ALBERT BANERJEE is a PhD candidate at York University, specializing in the sociology of health. He is concurrently completing a diploma in Health Services and Policy Research and holds an MA in Communications and a PhD in Psychology from Simon Fraser University. His current research includes an international comparative study of long-term care in Canada and Nordic Europe.

MARCY COHEN is the research and policy director of the Hospital Employees Union and a research associate with the B.C. Centre for Policy Alternatives. She has led several research studies on the implications of community health and long-term care restructuring in B.C. She has also co-authored a number of studies on the work environment, staffing, injury rates and ownership in long-term care.

NICOLE ESHKAKOGAN is a PhD student in Sociology at the University of Alberta, specializing in the sociology of death. She has extensive experience in research and evaluation, and has co-authored several articles in the area of Aboriginal aging and health. She has worked with provincial and federal Aboriginal health promotion programs, social service agencies and educational/training institutions.

NENE ERNEST KHALEMA is an assistant professor of Social Work at the University of Calgary. Khalema's research background is in social epidemiology, community-based research, health equity, immigrant/refugee integration and anti-oppression praxis. He has worked as a research coordinator and analyst for a number of academic institutions, not-for-profit agencies and community-based organizations in Alberta.

DICK MOORE is the coordinator of the Older LGBT (lesbian, gay, bisexual and transgender) program at Toronto's 519 Church Street Community Centre.

He provides leadership to the Senior Pride Network, a group committed to expanding programs and services for older LGBTs. Dick received the 2006 Access and Equity Award from the City of Toronto for his work.

SHEILA NEYSMITH is a professor in Social Work at the University of Toronto and director of the faculty's PhD program. She has published extensively on how policies affect the caring labour that women do throughout their lives. Her books include *Telling Tales: Living the Effects of Public Policy* and *Restructuring Caring Labour: Discourse, State Practice and Everyday Life*.

MORGAN SEELEY is a doctoral candidate in the school of Women's Studies at York University. She is also a member of the Women and Health Care Reform group. Inspired by feminist approaches to Critical Disability Studies, her thesis explores the experiences of young adults with disabilities living in institutional long-term care facilities in southern Ontario.

EVELYN SHAPIRO is a senior scholar in the Department of Community Health Sciences, Faculty of Medicine, at the University of Manitoba. A senior policy advisor to governments, she has published extensively on the determinants of health among the elderly and the impact of social policy on long-term institutional care. She is a member of the Order of Canada and the Order of Manitoba.

BEVERLY SUEK is co-chair of the Committee for Retirement Alternatives, exploring housing options for women. She has a history of working for women's equality in Manitoba and helped establish a women's housing cooperative, the Women's Enterprise Centre and the Immigrant Women's Employment Counselling Centre. As a management consultant she has worked with governments, unions, community-based groups and First Nations communities.

MARTA SZEBEHELY is a professor of Social Work at Stockholm University. Her fields of research include gender, social policy and care in historical and comparative perspectives in Scandinavia, Canada and Australia. She is responsible for research on care in aging and diversifying societies within the new Nordic Centre of Excellence: Reassessing the Nordic Welfare Model.

# Preface

Pat Armstrong

We have heard a great deal in recent years about the threat posed to our medical system by our "aging" population. For even longer, we have heard stories about the horrors of "being put in a home." Care at home is offered as the primary solution, and there is little talk about how to make residential care a positive option and a place for dignified care. This book is about promoting that conversation.

It is also about addressing long-term facility care as a woman's issue. Most of those who live in long-term care facilities are women, although more men have been joining them there in recent years as other kinds of institutional care are closed and as hospitals focus on narrowly defined acute care. Just as important, the overwhelming majority of those who work in residential care are women. Women are also the ones most likely to provide unpaid support in these facilities. Yet very little of the research and policy discussion on long-term care recognizes the importance of gender or of gender relations in long-term care facilities. This book brings a gender lens to the analysis.

In several ways, this collection is a result of the collaboration known as the Women and Health Care Reform Group. We are a multi-disciplinary group that investigates and advises on the effects of health care reforms on women as providers, decision-makers and users of health care systems. As part of the Women's Health Contribution Program of Health Canada's Bureau of Women's Health and Gender Analysis, our mandate is to coordinate research on health care reform and to translate this research into policies and practices. In all our work, we explore the issues for women, always asking which women are affected in what ways.

One way we carry out this mandate is by organizing workshops to bring those employed in policy and research together with health care practitioners. These workshops help to develop a better understanding of what the issues are for women and how these issues can be addressed in ways that take differences among women into account. One of these workshops focused on designing long-term residential care with women in mind.

Participants were sent two background documents to promote a shared basis for discussion. The conceptual paper I wrote with PhD student Albert Banerjee, "Challenging Questions," was intended to provoke debate and encourage participants to confront the assumptions we make about long-term residential care. Albert also undertook an overview of long-term care facilities in Canada because there is no place to go to find such a description.

The workshop began with a public forum. Stockholm-based professor and researcher Marta Szebehely developed a portrait of eldercare in Sweden, suggesting a social model as an alternative approach to residential services. In Sweden, not only are most services publicly provided and such care defined as a right but, as she explains in her article here, the government is under pressure to develop a gender-based analysis of eldercare. By way of contrast, Sheila Neysmith, a professor at the University of Toronto, examined the challenging situation of women and long-term care in Canada's most populous province, Ontario, and her article in this volume extends the comparison.

The rest of the chapters began as panel presentations and were later further developed by the authors and/or by our editor Jane Springer, integrating aspects of the workshop discussion.

We wanted the workshop to move beyond specific practices to principles. Presenters were asked to set the stage for the development of strategies that take into account women as residents, as paid and unpaid care providers, as decision-makers and as family members. We encouraged the panelists to help us think about what, in relation to its physical, cultural and social environments, makes facility care good for residents and for their families and providers.

In this book, Evelyn Shapiro and Morgan Seeley, advocates of publicly funded long-term care, begin the discussion with an impassioned exposure of what happens in private residential facilities. Nicole Eshkakogan, an Alberta researcher, sets out Aboriginal women's and men's long-term care needs within the changing context of their lives.

Based on her expertise as a union researcher and policy director in British Columbia, Marcy Cohen focuses on what women workers need in order to provide care that treats residents with dignity and respect. Dick Moore, coordinator of an Older Lesbian, Gay, Bisexual and Transgender program in Toronto, shares promising strategies for taking the interests of LGBT communities into account. Drawing on her experience as part of a diverse group of women who have defined exactly the type of facility and programming they want in long-term care, Beverly Suek addresses the obstacles to planning for our own later years.

These articles are not intended as definitive pieces, setting out the perfect blueprint for care. Nor are they meant to make decisive interventions. Rather they are thought-provoking essays to stimulate us all to start designing long-term care with women in mind, to begin imagining and prepare to realize a place we would be willing to call home.

# 1 Challenging Questions

## Designing Long-Term Residential Care with Women in Mind

Pat Armstrong with Albert Banerjee

Long-term residential care in Canada exists in the shadows, largely invisible in the debates on health care reform and rarely considered from a gendered perspective.

The *Canada Health Act*, the legislation that sets out the principles for our public health system, does not mention such care. The Romanow Report on the future of health care in Canada (2002) barely does. A 2006 Canadian Institute for Health Information (CIHI) publication on facility-based long-term care talks about presenting "an emerging portrait of a little-known sector" (CIHI 2006: iii). With data on voluntary reports from 7 out of 71 residential care facilities in Nova Scotia, it provides a very limited snapshot of the Canadian population in such care. Whitney Berta and colleagues (2006) offer a more comprehensive view based on Statistics Canada's annual national survey, the Residential Care Facilities Survey. They are able to produce a more complete picture of who owns and who resides in long-term care, show-ing the considerable variation across the country in the services provided. However, they are concerned that "policy around nature (sic) and quality of long-term care (LTC) for the future is virtually absent from the political agenda" (Berta et al. 2006: 176). It is not much of an issue for researchers, either. For example, while patient safety has become a major issue in hospitals, it has been largely ignored in long-term care (Castle et al. 2007). Nor has it received much attention at the international level. As the Organization for Economic Cooperation and Development points out, international estimates and profiles for long-term care are not well developed compared to other areas of public spending (Huber 2005). In short, long-term care is hardly at the centre of either research and data collection or policy debates.

Yet long-term care facilities are neither new nor destined for extinction in the near future. There have been such facilities in Canada for well over a century. They have primarily served the elderly but they also provide care for many younger people with severe disabilities. We can predict that the cultural mix of residents will change as the impact of immigration since the Second

World War plays out among the old (Statistics Canada 2007a). It is harder to predict the extent to which the post-war generation will need long-term care as the proportion of seniors in the population increases. Other factors, such as changes in marital practices and in fertility, greater geographical mobility and new technologies will also influence the profile of long-term care residents. But even with a considerable expansion in home care services, we can confidently predict that the demand for long-term residential care will not disappear in the near future. What is often called the "aging of the population" has not lacked for attention in policy circles. The focus, however, has been primarily on the costs rather than on the quality of care and on medical rather than on care needs. Disability, too, has received some policy attention in recent years, but almost all the attention has been on closing facilities rather than on the people who remain in such care.

We can also predict that gender will matter in long-term care, given that gender plays a role in all social relations and especially in care ones. Long-term care matters for women in particular because women account for the overwhelming majority of residents and of providers. Although federal government policy requires a gender-based analysis where appropriate, the Romanow report fails to provide it. Few of the other reports that focus on long-term care do either. The Canadian Institute for Health Information does note that women account for 71 percent of the residents in Nova Scotia long-term care facilities and that there are "three times more women than men in the 85 and older group" (CIHI 2006: 23). But the analysis stops there, without going on to explore any other aspects of gender in facility care or the factors that contribute to this distribution. For example, research from the United States indicating that men's experiences and behaviour in long-term care differ from women's suggests that the gender of residents is a relevant factor for analysis (Moss and Moss 2007).

Berta and colleagues look at staffing, but fail to even mention that women account for four out of five workers in these facilities and a significant proportion of the managers in long-term care (Armstrong, Armstrong and Scott-Dixon 2006). They also comment on the importance of "volunteer care" without considering the gendered nature of this volunteer care work and they have nothing to say about the gender of residents (Berta et al. 2006: 192). Yet research by Donna Baines (2004) shows that the unpaid labour in facilities is often provided by female workers who are also paid employees in that workplace. Such "volunteer" labour follows highly gendered lines, with men less likely than women to provide this unpaid overtime. Women are also much more likely than men to provide unpaid care to family and friends who live in facilities (Grant et al. 2004). Men do seem to be providing more care than in the past, especially to spouses, but they still lag behind women. And research in Quebec indicates that women may no longer be willing to take responsibility for unpaid care for family and friends, suggesting there may be growing opposition to providing this unpaid care (Guberman et al. 2006). In any case, the majority of women are now in paid employment, making it difficult for them to take on additional unpaid care work that may be required in the future. In other words, even though we have enough research to show that gender matters in terms of residents, providers, families and decision-making, a gender analysis is usually absent from the limited data and policy debate on long-term care.

Why is long-term care so poorly documented, analyzed and debated in the policy realm? And why is gender largely ignored in much of the policy and in many of the research documents that are available? In setting out some suggested factors below, we seek to set the stage for challenging these factors and for thinking through alternative approaches in long-term residential care, or in what may also be called nursing or personal care homes.

## Long-Term Care as Failure

As author, consultant and former professor Bruce Vladeck (2004: 2) puts it, long-term care is "something most people don't like to talk about; denial and avoidance are powerful psychological phenomena, especially in a society eager to promote the fantasy that no one really ever has to grow old." Such facilities, he says, have become institutions of last resort that emerge in response to problems in other social institutions (Vladeck 2003). While he is talking about the United States, it is equally the case in Canada and much the same thing could be said about long-term disability. Long-term care facilities are based on particular notions of care, of family, of individuals and of women. For the most part, LTC is riddled with notions of failure on the part of them all, even though these notions are rarely articulated and even more rarely linked. These are failures we would rather not think about.

In order to begin a discussion about what long-term residential care with women in mind would look like, it is important to unpack these notions and challenge some central assumptions. As Sylvia Tesh argued in the first edition of what has become a classic book (*Hidden Arguments: Political Ideology and Disease Prevention Policy*), we need to get these assumptions and "the politics out of hiding" before we can begin a process of transformation. Like the Romanow Report, Tesh holds that "we need public discussion about the values, beliefs, and ideologies with which scientists and policy-makers begin" (Tesh 1988: 6). Against this backdrop, it is possible to move towards the development of ideas and practices for long-term care in which it has its own mandate — not as a solution to failure, not as an institution of last resort, but as an essential, gender-sensitive public service responsive to diversity within caring communities.

## Hidden Assumptions about Care

In medical care, success is about treatment and cure. And, increasingly, it is about cure in a short period of time. Drugs, surgery and technologies are the main methods defining treatment in care. Hospitals are places for such care, with recent reforms focused on reducing hospital stays as much as possible. Over the last two decades, we have seen hospitals become more narrowly defined in ways that exclude much of the chronic and rehabilitative care once provided in places called hospitals. Indeed, CIHI distinguishes hospital-based continuing care from hospital care by saying that the "goal of care may not be cure," even though most of those admitted into continuing care stay less than three months (CIHI 2006: 2, 1).

This distinction is important for more than one reason. First, when people leave hospitals, they are now understood to be leaving the protection of the principles involved in the *Canada Health Act*. This lack of protection under the Act itself suggests that less value is attached to other forms of care and allows provinces/territories greater leeway in providing public services. Fees can be charged, means tests applied, services excluded and provincial/territorial barriers introduced. As soon as payment becomes a factor in access to care, women are more likely than men to be denied access because they are less likely to have paid jobs, because they earn less when they do work for pay, and because their paid jobs are less likely to come with supplementary health benefits or pensions. Moreover, women are less likely to remarry after a heterosexual marriage breaks down and therefore less likely to have a spouse to assist them financially in their old age. We have little information about what happens to women in old age who have been in same-sex relationships, but there are few reasons to believe they are better off financially than their heterosexual counterparts. Women often cannot afford the parts of care defined as extras, such as private rooms, or may not get in at all because only private rooms with extra costs are available or because their provincial government does not cover this care. These charges also reinforce differences among women, privileging those with access to financial resources.

Second, those who enter a long-term care facility are usually defined as beyond cure or significant improvement from medical methods and thus as a failure of medicine. As a resident told Rory Coughlan and Linda Ward, in their study of quality in long-term care in Ontario, "when you come in here, your former doctor gives up on you" (Coughlan and Ward 2007: 53). A majority of the people in these residential facilities have been labeled as having some form of dementia, itself often seen as incurable (CIHI 2006: 24). In fact, dementia combined with some other form of severe functional limitation seems increasingly to be a basic criterion for entry as it becomes harder to get into public residential care. This link with the other major neglected area in health services, namely mental health, may contribute to the low value and invisibility attached to long-term residential care. The fact that people leave the facility only for what are increasingly very short periods of intervention in hospitals reinforces the cure/incurable distinction. That most leave when they die reinforces the notion of failure, given that in medicine death is often defined that way — as it is more generally in our society.

The people who live in long-term care facilities are called residents and the facility is called a residence or even a home, further distinguishing the facilities from hospitals. Yet the residents are categorized primarily in terms of medical diagnosis. And both funding and staffing are assessed in relation to these diagnoses (Berta et al. 2006). Physically, the facility often looks like a hospital and is usually modelled on the hierarchies in hospital care. Public funding is often limited to medical interventions, and residents are charged for the accommodation costs that are supposed to make a facility a home (Sawyer and Stephenson 2002 [1995]). Moreover, care is usually divided up into specific, time-limited tasks reflecting a notion of people as body parts, with usually little recognition of the emotional and social support residents need as part of their care. Instead, efficiency and effectiveness are measured mainly in terms of the speed and quantity of tasks completed. Quality of care measurements are primarily medical, assessing such clinically related aspects as bed sores, falls, incontinence and restraint use. At the same time, many of the regulations and rules are aimed only at preventing the worst forms of abuse rather than at promoting a supportive, homelike environment (Gass 2004). On the basis of their Ontario research on long-term care, Coughlan and Ward conclude that these measures "are often impoverished and abstracted from the processes involved in care delivery and the environment in which they often occur, and lacking both sociopsychological aspects and the voices of patients." In contrast, the "residents understood 'quality of care' to be better defined as 'quality of life'" (Coughlan and Ward 2007: 48). The residents' definition seemed much closer to the notion of a residence or home than to practices based on medical measurements of quality.

There is a third reason for understanding the distinction between hospital and residential care facilities and the link to failure. Defining these services out of the main part of public medical care, and as an area where medicine can no longer succeed, has allowed provincial and territorial governments to promote long-term care provided by entrepreneurs searching for profit. Long-term care becomes defined as a service like any other, removing the claim to such care as a human right. This separation allows for the recent rapid development of residential care services that are for purchase, and that in most jurisdictions lack the kind of regulation applied to other care services. Although they do not receive direct public funding, they do not receive public scrutiny either. Equally important, they separate those with funding from those without, leaving only people with no alternative seeking subsidized public care. It suggests a return to long-term care as poorhouses, houses where women dominate as a result of their lack of resources in old age.

Important here too is the notion that public health services have failed to be as efficient and effective as the private, for-profit sector and that competition will lead to better choice as well as to cheaper services. Such an assumption promotes competitive bidding for government care contracts, government payments to for-profit firms and the adoption within public facilities of practices taken from the for-profit sector. A host of research is starting to reveal problems with the assumption of for-profit superiority, as well as with the assumption that for-profit methods are appropriate for care. Staffing levels in for-profit facilities tend to be lower than in non-profit ones; more of the care is provided by those with the least formal training; hospital admissions are higher from these facilities and so are formal complaints. Competitive bidding may not only increase instability and promote the minimum of care but also reduce both voluntary sector participation and resident choice (Berta et al. 2006). Ownership and market principles also raise questions about decision-making and stability. With many large owners in the health-care field and managers responsible to shareholders, local control may well be lost. Stability too may be at risk because for-profit firms will close if their facility is no longer profitable (McKay 2003b; Cloutier-Fisher and Skinner 2006; McGrail et al. 2007; McGregor et al. 2005; Shapiro and Tate 1995).

There is an additional point to be made about the value put on medical intervention and the contrasting value attached to long-term care. Workers in hospitals are more highly valued than those in long-term care. This value difference is evident in their wages and benefits as well as in the extent of their formal training. According to Berta and colleagues, those living in long-term care need "high levels of daily personal care entailing supervision or assistance with activities of daily living, 24 hour nursing care or supervision, and a secure environment" (Berta et al. 2006: 177). The registered nurses and licensed practical nurses who work in long-term care usually meet the same educational requirements as nurses in hospitals and may even have specialized training in geriatric care. But they are usually paid less than their hospital counterparts (Armstrong and Laxer 2006). Most of the care, however, is provided by personal care providers, who may or may not have formal education and who are not well paid for the work. Many of them have credentials, and most have become highly skilled at their jobs through long experience (Armstrong and Daly 2004). The failure to require credentials and training, though, reflects the idea that assistance with daily living does not require many skills. Equally important, it is assumed any woman can do such work by virtue of being a woman and it is mainly women who do the personal care work. Indeed, women make up a higher percentage of this workforce than they do in the overall health care sector. This is women caring for women, a factor that may also contribute to the value associated with the facilities, the residents and the workers.

The point is not that medical or clinical care should be eliminated from long-term care. Rather, it is that we need to explore the implications of the dominance of the medical model in our approach to long-term care. And we need to examine the relationship between this model and assumptions about gender, drawing out the consequences for the construction of care and care work within residences.

## Hidden Assumptions about Families

Introducing a journal issue on family and aging, Francis Caro claims that "the emergence of public interventions to address special needs of elders can be traced to the limitations of families" (Caro 2006: 1). Similar claims are made about younger people in facility care. The implication is that families have failed, either because there is no one left or because they refuse to fulfill their obligations to provide care as families did in the past. In any case, it sets up public care as the last choice, a poor alternative. And what we usually mean by families is female relatives, although we do expect male spouses to do more than they did twenty years ago and do expect men to provide financial support. The notion of family failure can add to the guilt and concern women feel as relatives, as well as to the hesitation they have in considering sending their relatives into long-term care unless every other possibility is exhausted, including their own health. This, in turn, contributes to the notion of long-term care as a last resort. So does the kind of investigation that happens before someone is admitted to a public long-term care facility. You have to prove considerable need and, increasingly, no family alternative before you are allowed public support for long-term residential care.

Yet the claim that families, and the women in them, now fail in comparison to the past does not stand up to scrutiny (Armstrong and Kitts 2004). There is a long history of paid providers in private households and plenty of evidence that people went without care. We have no strong evidence that most families or even the women in them have throughout history provided the kinds of care required in long-term facilities today. Nor do we have much evidence on the quality of care that was provided in families and by women. We mainly assume it was adequate, without investigation. Adequacy seems to be defined as what women did to provide care, whatever that was, and it was assumed that everyone lived in families with women who could provide care. The assumption that women are not providing the kind of care their mothers did for the elderly and disabled in the past is largely without basis in the research.

Moreover, there are several important differences between the current situation and that in the past. A much higher proportion of the population is surviving with severe functional limitations, and a significantly greater proportion of the population is living into very old age, thus increasing the demand on families for care. Sophisticated medical techniques can now be used in the home, permitting the kinds of care there that were never possible in the past. The fertility rate has fallen and family members are more geographically mobile, leaving fewer children to provide care for those with high needs. Divorce is more common and more women than men are left without partners in their old age. In the past, many women died at an early age from childbirth and thus fewer lived to need long-term care. The majority of women have now joined the majority of men in the labour force and most of their adult children have paid jobs. Both women and men work for similar reasons, even though women still retain the primary responsibility for domestic tasks. This leaves few people at home to provide more complex care, except for other people who are elderly or disabled and who often have their own heavy care needs.

Nevertheless, there is little evidence to suggest families in general, or women in particular, have abandoned their relatives and sent them into long-term care as the demands on their time and for their care labour increase. Rather, there is plenty of evidence that women have sacrificed their own health and labour force careers to provide long-term care and to avoid sending their relatives into facilities. There has been no growth in the proportion of the elderly and severely disabled in residential long-term care, even though their numbers have increased significantly and public services have been withdrawn. As women, and some men, make these sacrifices to provide care, they further reinforce the notion that residential, public care is the last resort.

Nor is there evidence that women fail to provide care once their relatives become residents in long-term facilities. Research from Quebec suggests that both women and men remain committed to supporting family members who need care, and that this is particularly the case for spouses. Perhaps surprisingly, people between the ages of 18 and 30 felt more strongly about family responsibility than older respondents (Guberman et al. 2006). This may bode well for the future. Nevertheless, this research also suggests that all age groups and both women and men are open to formal services. Their support does not necessarily mean they want to provide direct, personal care. Within Canada, there are cultural variations in the extent to which women and other family members say they are committed to provide long-term care for their relatives, although there is less variation in the actual care provided. There are also class variations in the extent to which families in general and women in particular can support their relatives by paying for care. In all cultures, women feel the primary responsibility for personal care.

Family commitment may not be enough, however. The location of facilities, especially when combined with government policies that limit choices in terms of residences, may mean families find it difficult to provide care to relatives in long-term facilities. This is especially a problem for women, who are more likely to rely on public transit, and for those who live in rural areas without public transit. Poor women and women who live alone are particularly likely to rely on such means to get to facilities or even homes to provide care. Similarly, workplace policies can limit the possibilities for combining support in facilities or other forms of unpaid care with paid employment. Given that women's paid jobs tend to be more precarious than those of men, women may find it even more difficult to keep up their support once relatives enter care facilities (Vosko 2006).

The recent emphasis in policy on home care also reinforces the notion that families have failed when relatives become residents in long-term care. As Nancy Guberman explains on the basis of her extensive research on home care in Quebec, families are represented as characterized by warmth, love, spontaneity, freedom and flexibility while institutions are represented as cold, professional, unfeeling, inflexible and regimented. "Therefore, despite the numerous documented difficulties of caring and being cared for at home, this appears to be the only real choice available" (Guberman 2004). At the same time, as her more recent research with Quebec colleagues shows, most people do not want their families to provide their personal care and few family members "would freely and willingly choose to do so" (Guberman et al. 2006: 74). Those with financial resources can afford to create their own options but many women do not have the resources to either buy the care they need or to pay someone to provide the care others need. Given that women have more limited financial resources than men and that women are more likely to need and provide care, this is particularly an issue for women.

The point here is not that families should not or will not provide care to those with long-term care needs; nor is it that men should simply take on half of the care work. Rather, it is that we need to examine the assumptions we make about family care and explore the consequences for women as providers and as those who need care.

## Hidden Assumptions about Individual Failure

Too often entry into long-term care is defined not only as a failure of families but also as a failure of the individual. Independence has long been highly valued in much of our society, and in recent years there has been even greater stress on taking responsibility for our own health. Increasingly in public policy, we assume that ideal citizens take care of themselves. As Eva Feder Kittay, an internationally recognized scholar on disability, eloquently puts it, "we are captives of the myth of the independent, unembodied subject — not born, not developing, not ill, not disabled and never growing old — that dominates our thinking about matters of justice and questions of policy" (Kittay et al. 2005: 445). According to Canadian disability activist and lawyer David Shannon, "the disabled person is considered an object to be pitied because he or she could neither fit into a society mainstream nor care for his or herself" (Shannon 2007: 1). Long-term care is necessarily about dependency in at least some aspects of care. In such an environment, long-term care is frequently seen as failure on the part of the individual to protect their health and to provide for their own care.

Our notions of dependency have changed over time and remain highly gendered. The ideal of dependency has, in the dominant Canadian society at least, been mainly about men and most often associated with Caucasian ones. It has been acceptable for women to be dependent on men for protection from many threats and for financial support. However, women have been expected to provide the bulk of care in return for this protection. Dependency on others for care has not been acceptable for women either. And increasingly women are expected to be financially independent as well. The current policies on mothers seeking welfare provide just one example of the expectation that women should not depend on the government for financial support even when their children are young (Little 1998).

As is the case with ideas about family responsibility, notions of independence also vary with culture and physical location. Among Aboriginal people, for instance, the "circle is used to represent the inseparability of the individual from their family, community and the world.... This interconnectedness is an integral philosophical concept that was common to many different Aboriginal people who lived throughout North America" (Prokop et al. 2004: 149–50). It is a concept that is hard to maintain within a dominant culture that stresses independence while failing to create the conditions that would allow most Aboriginal people to be either individually independent or self-sufficient within their interdependent communities. In other words, while alternative perspectives on independence exist, they are neither dominant nor supported.

Dependency in the short term is not usually understood as failure. As sociologist Talcott Parsons explained years ago, sick people are allowed to be dependent when they are defined as ill but are expected to work hard at getting better so they can return to independence (Parsons 1951). Children are expected to become increasingly independent as they grow, and disabled people are expected to struggle to manage on their own. The emphasis is often on entry or return to the labour force, given that labour force work is understood as the primary basis of independence and of contribution to society. However, those in long-term care residences are not going to return to paid work and the women are not going back to providing unpaid domestic services for their families.

This value placed on independence, combined with a medical model of care, contributes to the notion of individual failure on the part of those in long-term care. No longer independent in some aspects, residents may be defined as incapable of independence in all aspects. This may help explain why many residents in Ontario nursing homes "felt a sharp distinction between their previously independent lives whereas now, they reported that they often felt they are merely a list of tasks for staff to attend to" (Coughlan and Ward 2007: 52). Defined as dependent and thus as failing at the goal of independence, they may no longer be allowed independence of any sort. These notions of failure linked to dependency may also support a managerial and policy emphasis on counting and measuring tasks in ways that focus on the job and not on the person needing care.

Ideas about the importance of independence, then, are problematic for two reasons. First, they can mean those who are dependent are not highly valued and the value attached to independence may be different for women and for men. Second, it can mean that those defined as dependent are denied any independence and are without rights to claim such independence in any aspects of their lives. This, in turn, contributes to the emphasis on tasks and on long-term care facilities as not a place where life continues but as a place to wait, often understood as waiting for the end (Coughlan and Ward 2007). Whether there are gender differences in these attitudes is not explored in the research but should be a question for investigation.

## Alternative Patterns: Contradictory Notions

Of course, not everyone sees long-term facility care as a symbol of failure on the part of medicine, families, women and/or individuals. Many of those who live and work in facilities, and of those who have friends or families living in them, do not share this view of long-term residences as symbols of failure. Some managers and policy-makers work hard to counter this perspective and to build an alternative perspective. As Vladeck puts it, some facilities work "remarkably well," and when they do, usually the reason "is the energy, dedication, compassion, and creativity of the primary caregivers — the nursing home and home care aides, nursing assistants and personal care workers" (Vladeck 2004: 3).

Nevertheless, failure is a prevalent view. And it is a view that contributes to the low visibility of long-term facility care on policy agendas, to the burden families and especially the women in them carry, and to the way individual women are treated in care. These views are realized in the structures and processes of care. Equally important, there are those who see long-term care in facilities as necessarily bad and therefore something that should be abolished rather than analyzed with a view to making care there better for everyone.

However, if we want to make long-term facility care a priority on the health care reform agenda, we have to deal with these often hidden assumptions. We have to expose and debate them in order to lay the foundations for fundamental reforms in long-term care. Questions of access cannot be addressed without challenging the notion of failure on the part of families and the women in these families. Questions about the kind of care provided, along with the processes and people involved, cannot be addressed without challenging the notion of failure on the part of the medical model and the ideas about women's work. Questions about alternatives to long-term care cannot be addressed without challenging the notion of individual failure and dependency. These notions in turn must be related not only to gender but also to differences among women and among men.

## Challenging Premises: Raising Questions

Challenging the notion of long-term facility care as failure requires more than an exposure of the hidden assumptions that too often guide our policy and practices. It also requires the identification of different premises about care, dependency and families. And it requires a gender analysis that goes well beyond the analysis of data by sex to relate long-term residential care to the reality of women's lives and to differences among women. With alternative premises, it is possible to move towards gender-sensitive practices for organizing and delivering long-term care. There are no simple formulas for moving away from current assumptions, for developing alternative ones or for transforming principles into practices. The following is intended as a starting point for discussion, a way of framing debates rather than settling them.

### Dependency and the Individual

To move towards designs for long-term care with women in mind, we have to change our view of those who need personal care and need support with aspects of daily living. And tackling the notion of individual failure means tackling the very idea of independence and individual responsibility. Although Western liberal thought has long stressed the importance of self-reliance, interdependency is part of the human condition. We vary significantly in the extent of our capacities and contributions, but we necessarily depend on others for food, clothing, shelter, jobs and joy. The dependency that may come with old age and with disability does differ from other forms in that it often requires personal, intimate kinds of care for people unable to manage aspects of daily maintenance alone. But this too is part of the human condition, a part we accept in infancy but too often reject at older ages. But even in infancy, we usually see this dependency as the private responsibility of the mother especially, and not part of our collective responsibility as a caring society.

A different approach to long-term residential care involves different notions of dependency and of collective responsibility for care. It begins with the recognition that we have a universal right to care, which involves an understanding of care that goes beyond the narrow confines of medical intervention. As Kittay so neatly puts it, an "ethic of care regards dependence as a central feature of human life and human relationships and interdependency rather than independence as a goal in human development" (Kittay et al. 2005: 453).

From this perspective, failure is then defined as our collective failure to provide care for dependent individuals in ways that recognize their capacities as well as their limitations. Starting from this premise raises significant questions both about access to care and about how care is structured. Approaching the question with women in mind also requires an investigation of the nature and conditions of women's lives in and outside residential care.

If we start with the principles of the *Canada Health Act* as it applies to hospitals, we can then ask how to make residential care accessible to women in ways that remove financial and other barriers. Charges for entry limit women's access more than men's, given women's lower income and pensions, and charges limit some women's access more than others. Within residences, charges for services that are essential to dignity and support create barriers for women as well. Reducing barriers thus means providing comprehensive services without charges, services that would include necessary ones like room, board, haircuts and outings. But financial barriers go well beyond actual costs. Means tests, based on assessments of economic worth to determine eligibility, are another indication of the way we view the right to care and individual failure. Women are more likely than men to meet the means tests and qualify for assistance but at what costs to their personal dignity and right to care? Physical location can also constitute a barrier if women can no longer relate to the people, places and activities where they have established their identities. Cultural barriers such as the nature of the food provided as well as the times the food is provided and the way it is delivered are also important, as are language barriers. Indeed, being placed in facilities that operate with cultural and language practices that are alien to the resident can make residents appear more disabled than they are and even promote decline.

Access thus also means having options among and within facilities. This, in turn, implies diversity not only in the location but also in the structure and organization of residential facilities as well as access to care services in the home. For example, research in the United States indicates that residents in specialized dementia care units were more involved in activities, took fewer drugs and were less likely to be incontinent than those in general facilities. And their care providers were more likely to have specialized training and to be satisfied with their jobs (Robinson and Pillemer 2007). Women-only residences might also prove to be an attractive alternative. Of course, we cannot provide endless options for everyone but we can balance demands with a wider range of possibilities.

Lack of integration among services may be equally important in limiting access, but too much integration may also mean there is only one option for long-term residential care. If you fail to qualify at the single entry point, for example, you may be denied admission to any publicly funded facility. We need to have means of determining what kinds of integration work for both providers and for those who need care, and then put the research into practice. A care management scheme for the elderly in Quebec was effective at reducing hospitalization and improving access to health and social services. It also helped improve care provider satisfaction, but we do not know how the elderly assessed this strategy and it was an experiment that did not receive continuing funding (Kodner 2006). In short, barriers can be gender-specific and can extend beyond the obvious financial and physical ones.

Challenging notions of dependency means challenging more than questions related to who gets into facilities on what basis. It also means altering the way we see dependency and the way people who are dependent are treated. Dependency in some aspects of daily life does not necessarily mean total incapacity or dependency in all aspects of life, yet there is often the tendency to treat residents this way. Research suggests that residents who have more autonomy and control are not only in better health but also rely less on supportive services and participate more actively in residence life (Sikorska-Simmons 2006a). U.S. research suggests that non-profit facilities are more likely than for-profit ones to offer flexibility in scheduling and possibilities for participation (Moos and Lemke 1994). In a rare study that interviewed residents themselves, Coughlan and Ward found residents using toileting as an example of dependency and dignity. Without enough staff to help residents maintain bladder control, residents worried about participating in activities where they might lose control and thus spent more time alone. They often became more incontinent and felt pressured to turn to diapers (Coughlan and Ward 2007). This dependency, in turn, had a negative impact on their feeling of self-worth. Women who have given birth may be particularly at risk of losing bladder control or of worrying about whether they will. Unfortunately, we do not know from this study, or from many others, if there are gender differences in the ways women and men see indicators of dignity and self-worth or even bladder control issues, although it is clearly an important question in planning for care.

The Eden Alternative, a U.S. approach to long-term facility care, starts with the assumption that most suffering by residents is caused by loneliness, boredom and helplessness (Lopez 2006). The question then becomes, how can we provide opportunities to utilize their full capacities in ways that reflect residents' particular histories and culture? And how can we do this in ways that recognize the gendered patterns of their lives and build on their experience? For example, some facilities offer cooking classes. However, places to cook may be a better alternative because kitchens would be based on the assumption women already know how and would like to use their skills. But women do much more than cook in their daily lives, so it is important to involve them in ways that allow them to demonstrate as well as use their full range of current skills that go well beyond those associated with traditional women's work.

Small and large schemes are required. On the basis of his participant observation in three U.S. facilities, Steven Lopez offers one small strategy designed to transform our views of residents in a facility for the elderly. Each room has a picture of the resident when they were young. The picture serves not only to remind providers that residents had lives outside the residence that were much like their own but also to reveal how many residents see themselves and to provide a basis for conversation (Lopez 2006). Other strategies are required to recognize differences in cultural practices and to create conditions for following familiar patterns with dignity. So too are strategies to allow residents a say in their care and to involve their families as well.

In sum, challenging notions of individual failure means addressing more than issues of access, broadly defined. It also means changing the organization of care and social relations within facilities in ways that promote as much independence as possible without denigrating dependency in the process. It means recognizing that there are important gender and cultural differences in interests and capacities but doing so in ways that do not assume traditional gender divisions.

## Medical Models and Social Care

There is no shortage of challenges to the medical model, with its emphasis on fixing body parts through intervention by experts based on scientific evidence. Indeed, long-term care residences are defined as outside medicine even though they are organized and evaluated in medical terms. The challenge is to develop alternative models that understand success as quality of living and that value not only the residents but also those who provide their care. It would be a model that incorporates medicine but that also promotes dignity and respect by recognizing the context of individual lives, the contributions and skills of providers, and the importance of social relations as well as of social meanings. Translating models into practice represents an additional challenge.

A starting point is an emphasis on care as a relationship. This, in turn, implies several things. First, it means recognizing the importance of relationships and of building relationships with residents. What Lopez calls "organized emotional care" requires managers who not only value relationships but organize work in a manner that encourages such relationships (Lopez 2006). In the facility he observed where care was understood as a relationship, all workers were provided with opportunities to establish them. In this facility, the best housekeeper was "not the most efficient cleaner but rather one who was best at developing caring relationships with residents" (Lopez 2006). This approach contrasted sharply with the residence where the emphasis was on professional divisions among workers and professional distance from residents. In the latter case, both residents and providers were dissatisfied with care.

An emphasis on care as a relationship sensitive to women's diverse needs means a change in the culture and management of long-term care residences. However, this requires much more than training staff in cultural differences and providing rewards for the non-instrumental aspects of care, although these are clearly important. Cultural change means understanding the ways the medical model is reinforced by managerial practices taken from the for-profit sector, by a focus on short-term costs for governments and facilities, and by a notion that one size fits all. Understanding current practices within a context of the larger economy and of social relations can help us move towards strategies to change structures and policies that give primacy to medical approaches to long-term care.

Equally important are conditions that allow residents to develop relationships with other residents and with families. Coughlan and Ward found that residents often had their relationships with others in the facility disrupted by room changes that moved them away from roommates. Social relations were also made difficult by short periods for meals and disrupted encounters in other places where residents could interact (Coughlan and Ward 2007). Sexual relations and opportunities for couples to be alone may be prevented by the way residences are organized physically and socially. Such relations may also be impeded by the managers' or others' attitudes about sex among the elderly and/or about homosexuality.

Similarly, the way visits are organized and the spaces available for families have a significant impact on whether families can and want to visit. Poor care, or what appears to be poor care, can also discourage families from visiting because they often feel guilty about a situation over which they have little control. We do not have much research on how interactions in facilities differ by gender but we do have research suggesting that women and men value and form friendships in different ways, suggesting that gender-specific strategies to support relationships may be in order.

The second implication of starting with an understanding of care as a relationship has to do with the value we place on the work of those who provide care. A social model of care implies both understanding health in terms much broader than clinical interventions and developing skills that involve treating whole people in the context of their own histories and circumstances. Most of those who work in long-term care facilities are called personal care providers and many do the work without formal training, although not without skills. The long association of caring with women contributes to the idea both that the work is unskilled and that women know how to do it by virtue of being women, rather than as a result of learning. The low value attached to care work is reinforced by a lack of formal training. It is reinforced as well by the large number of women from racialized groups and from immigrant communities who themselves are often undervalued as workers. In turn, this low value contributes to the emphasis on care as a set of measured, timed tasks that managers can control and divide up among any women available to do the work.

Research in Canada and abroad shows that the work environment for staff sets the conditions for care. Residents are more satisfied and healthier when the staff is satisfied. The staff is more likely to be satisfied when there is more team work and participation in decision-making, when they have some autonomy in doing their work and when there are sufficient staff to provide the care they see as necessary (Coughlan and Ward 2007; Sikorska-Simmons 2006b; Tyler et al. 2006). And the level of staffing and of formal training is likely to be higher in non-profit facilities than in for-profit ones (McGregor et al. 2005; Shapiro and Tate1995). Equally important, relationships can only develop if the staff has secure, regular and long-term employment. Yet a large proportion of those employed in long-term care have precarious jobs and often hold more than one job in order to make a living wage. In other words, starting with care as a relationship means valuing the workers who support those relationships and providing them with the kinds of conditions and training that allows such relationships.

It also means developing alternative ways to assess care in facilities. The emphasis on medical indicators such as bed sores as a measure of quality should at least be supplemented by other measures that both assess and allow the relational aspects of care. It would mean evaluating safe environments in terms of the extent to which they support quality of life rather than mainly in terms of the use of drugs and restraints. It would mean consulting the residents, rather than assuming all of them are incapable of evaluating their care and conditions. It would mean consulting their families as well.

In sum, challenging the notion of long-term residential care as a medical failure means establishing an alternative model and then translating this into practices through different means of organizing work and of evaluating care. This too requires a gender perspective, given that the evaluation of the care work involved reflects the gendered divisions of care work.

## Family Resources

Challenging the association of long-term residential care with family failure means recognizing our shared, public responsibility for care. It also means challenging the notion that women are natural caregivers with a responsibility to provide a wide range of personal care services.

This does not mean that families should not or would not provide the kind of emotional and social support that the research by Guberman and colleagues show they want to provide (Guberman et al. 2006). Rather, it means creating the conditions that allow all family members, as well as friends, to provide the kind of support they want to provide. As mentioned earlier, the location and organization of facilities set the conditions for support by family and friends. If families are to provide support for those in residential care, then the facilities need to be family-friendly and to recognize that women in particular rely on public transit. Moreover, allowing women options both in terms of home care support and in terms of a range of facilities may reduce the guilt factor for both those who need care and those who provide care. Genuine options will only exist if good, public care is available in both the home and the facility.

The conditions for family care are not restricted to the conditions in facilities. With almost as many women as men employed in the labour force, the conditions of work are also important. As more and more people stay in the labour force past the age of 65, fewer of them will be available to provide unpaid care. However, women are more likely than men to have precarious work that may be put at risk by their efforts to provide support for relatives in long-term care. This requires the identification of policies that would allow both women and men to combine their paid jobs with support for family and friends in long-term care facilities.

What is required for family support, then, is better and more accessible care in long-term facilities as well as better conditions at work that would allow them to provide support to others. This requires recognition of the very different patterns in men's and women's daily lives, as well as differences among women in terms of resources and capacities.

## Summary

This chapter is intended to prompt and frame a discussion about what good residential care would look like for women. It begins by exposing and challenging the hidden assumptions about care, families, individuals and women, because such assumptions shape not only the way care is constructed and delivered but also access to care. It assumes that such care is both possible and necessary. While there are many who reject these assumptions, there can be no real choice for families, for workers and for individuals unless good, accessible facility care is available. This, in turn, requires us to figure out what good care would look like for women from different social, physical and economic locations. And it requires strategies on how to create or replicate such care. It also requires us to think in terms of gender and of gender relations, not only because women account for the overwhelming majority of residents and care providers but also because gender shapes the very process of care and the value we put on care.

There are innovative ideas in the current literature on long-term residential care. There are also practices worth replicating. But most of this literature lacks a gender analysis and even fewer of the practices begin with women in mind. So there is a great deal of room for new ideas about principles and practices and for ones that are gender-sensitive. How we construct long-term residential care that provides real options for women as residents and as providers — ones that recognize women's diversity as well as their shared needs — remains an open question.

# 2

# Long-Term Care in Canada

## An Overview

Albert Banerjee

This chapter is intended to provide a snapshot of long-term care in Canada. It begins with a brief discussion of the national context, followed by an outline of long-term care in several provinces (Nova Scotia, Ontario, Manitoba and British Columbia) and one territory (Yukon) in order to illustrate the diversity of long-term care across the country. A word of caution before beginning: the idea of "long-term care in Canada" is somewhat misleading. It lends a sense of concreteness and congruence that does not exist. Long-term care has different developmental histories in each province and territory, leading to a varied set of present circumstances. What's more, while Statistics Canada has been gathering data on residential care since 1974, there are few pan-Canadian analyses of long-term care, making any conversation at the national level a challenge.

This information deficit is starting to be addressed. For instance, the Canadian Institute for Health Information (CIHI) has embarked on a project to provide standardized information across Canadian provinces and territories. The first phase of this project resulted in a report released in 2006, *Facility-Based Continuing Care in Canada, 2004–2005* (CIHI 2006). However, to date, this report only covers the provinces of Ontario and Nova Scotia. Furthermore, as the Ontario sample is drawn from hospital-based continuing care facilities, it is not what some people mean when they ask about "long-term care." And in Nova Scotia, the sample only includes seven of the 71 long-term care facilities. Thus, confident statements about long-term care in Canada — such as the claim that 5 percent of residents are under the age of 65 — need to be taken with a grain of salt.

Another recent study draws on Statistics Canada data to provide a national portrait (Berta et al. 2006). However, as a result of differences in reporting style, Quebec is omitted from the picture, as are the territories. Indeed, it is a challenge to find any analysis comparing Quebec or the territories with other provinces. The report further groups the Prairie Provinces and the Atlantic Provinces in its analysis. This is problematic for a number of reasons. Not only is considerable information lost, but more importantly, in terms of understanding the organization and development of long-term care, provincial policy differences may well trump geography. Nonetheless, this study is a good beginning and this overview owes much to it.

Speaking about long-term care in the Canadian context is further complicated by the lack of a common language. Not only have national comparators not been established, but given the differing patterns of historical development, the formation of long-term care facilities, their function and their role in relation to other care institutions are somewhat location-specific. Thus, across jurisdictions, similarly named facilities do not necessarily provide similar services. For instance the CIHI (2006) report examines "residential facility based care" by which it means "nursing homes." Yet in Nova Scotia "residential care facilities" are not nursing homes at all. They are institutions offering intermediate levels of care more akin to the type of care provided in what Nova Scotians call "community based options" or what people in other provinces, such as Ontario, might term "supportive housing." Such differences in terminology can lead to confusion. And certainly caution is warranted. In assessing any national portrait, one does well to keep in mind the concern (if not frustration) expressed by the Federal/Provincial/Territorial Working Group on Home Care. In their words: "Review of available information revealed that there is hardly a statistic or description that would not be misleading or inaccurate without lengthy and complicated elaboration of its nuances, special circumstances, or unique meaning in a provincial or territorial context" (1990; quoted in Alexander 2002: 26).

## What is Long-Term Care?

Long-term care typically refers to ongoing, indefinite care for individuals who can no longer fully care for themselves. Long-term care straddles both *health care* in the form of nursing/medical care and *social services* in the form of income-supported housing, assistance with "activities of daily living" (i.e., basic functional tasks performed on a daily basis, such as general mobility, being able to clothe or feed oneself, to be continent and use the toilet, and to shower or bathe), and the provision of recreational and social programs (Vladeck 2003). Long-term care in Canada is commonly defined as representing

> a range of services that addresses the health, social and personal care needs of individuals who, for one reason or another, have never developed or have lost some capacity for self-care. Services may be continuous or intermittent, but it is generally presumed that they will be delivered for the "long-term" that is, indefinitely to individuals who have demonstrated need, usually by some index of functional incapacity. (F/P/T Subcommittee 1988, quoted in Havens 2002)

This overview is oriented by a notion of "long-term care" as referring to facilities that provide indefinite care for the elderly. Not all residents of long-term care facilities are elderly, as noted above. However, in many provinces separate facilities are provided for children and young adults; the idea is that while their health care needs may be similar, their social and recreational needs are not. Such facilities and individuals are not the focus of this chapter.

## Long-Term Care as Continuing Care

Long-term care is also commonly used to denote *continuing forms of care*. As such, it may refer to hospital-based continuing care, which generally tends to be more intense, complex and of shorter duration than long-term residential care. It may also be used to refer to home care or assisted living arrangements that provide basic levels of support and assume that the elderly are independently mobile and do not require 24-hour nursing care.

While neither continuing hospital care nor home care are the focus of this chapter, it is helpful to bear in mind that long-term care facilities for the elderly exist in the context of a *continuum of care* (Hollander 2002). Indeed, the "continuum of care" concept is gaining momentum in policy-making, as all levels of government are striving to better meet community needs, eradicate redundancies and increase efficiencies through the integration and coordination of services. With typical mission statement zeal, one often reads of the aim to provide "the right services, in the right place, at the right time" (Alexander 2002). More practically, the concept of a continuum of care reminds us that long-term care facilities *relate* to other institutions such as home care, assisted living, supportive housing, chronic care and complex continuing hospital-based care.

The continuum of care model thus has many implications for long-term care facilities. Decisions, for instance, around resource allocation and the building of new long-term care facilities are often made in relation to other institutions, in order to materially construct a continuum of care. At present, this appears to result in the allocation of funds away from long-term care facilities, towards home care, assisted living and other modes of keeping residents out of institutions and in the "community." Similarly, most jurisdictions have moved to single entry point systems in order to implement the continuum of care ideal at the individual level. Once again, as Pitters (2002) notes, a bias toward community care is built into intake assessment models. This means that assessment practice attempts to exhaust community care options before long-term care facilities are even considered. Whether or not this bias is sensitive to the needs of the elderly (and their informal caregivers) is an open question, but what appears clear is that when they do enter long-term care they are older and have greater health care needs. Long-term care also exists in relation to hospitals. The goal of shortening hospital stays, for instance, has resulted in the downloading of patients into long-term care facilities and the development, in some instances, of long-term sub-acute care beds. This has increased the number of residents with complex health care needs and has affected, not least, staff workloads and training requirements (OHC 2008).

## The Federal Policy Context

At present, long-term care — as institutionalized elderly care — is practically invisible at the federal level. The Romanow Report (2002), for instance, scarcely mentions long-term care. Two reasons are indicated in the report for this absence. On the one hand, the report privileges home care over long-term institutional care, the assumption being that residing in the home is more desirable and more cost effective than institutional care. However, priority home care services are limited in the report to mental health, palliative care and post acute services. Specific services for the elderly do not appear as a priority area. On the other hand, there is concern that institutionalized long-term care does not offer the flexibility required to respond to shifting population demographics and errors in demand forecasting. As Romanow explains: "Because it may be impossible to accurately forecast the health needs of the population too far in advance.... flexible approaches need to be taken to avoid the trap of investing in facilities and programs that may or may not be needed as Canada's population ages" (23).

Long-term care does not fall under the *Canada Health Act*. It therefore remains outside of the universally insured health services (Alexander 2002). In the past, the federal government provided targeted funding for long-term care through its Extended Health Care Services program (EHCS). Through this program money was transferred to provinces for long-term care facilities. Funding levels were set at $20 per capita when the program was established in 1977, an amount that had risen to $51.51 per capita by the early 1990s or a total of $1.5 billion annually in 1994–1995. Despite such growth, federal transfers for extended health care services were dwarfed by transfers for health services insured by the *Canada Health Act*. The EHCS program was abolished in 1996 with the introduction of the Canada Health and Social Transfer (CHST). The CHST collapsed federal transfers to the provinces for health, postsecondary education and welfare, thus eliminating targeted federal funding for long-term institutional care.

The federal government continues to have a hand in long-term care through its funding of First Nations' and Inuit's community care and veterans' long-term care.

## First Nations and Inuit Home and Community Care

Through Health Canada's First Nations and Inuit Home and Community Care (FNIHCC) program, the federal government provides assistance to First Nations and Inuit people across Canada (Health Canada 2004). The program is open to First Nations and Inuit people who live on a reserve (or North of 60 in a First Nations community) or in an Inuit settlement. The program receives approximately $90 million dollars annually and is available in over 600 communities across Canada. FNIHCC provides funding for home care services — including funding for non-medical personal care services such as meal preparation, light housekeeping, respite care and minor home mainte-nance. Of course, home care requires adequate homes, so it should be noted that in 2000–2001, only 55.8 percent of homes on First Nations reserves were considered to be adequate (FNIH 2007). Approximately 15 percent were in need of major repairs, and 5 percent were no longer habitable or had been declared unfit for human habitation.

The FNIHCC program also provides funding for institutional care. In 2002–2003, approximately $36 million was spent on long-term institutional care. However, FNIHCC funding only covers lower levels of care (Type 1 and Type 2 in the federal classification system, which refer to care requirements of less than two hours per day). This care is provided through provincial or territorial institutions (Health Canada 2004). The failure to provide funding for higher levels of care is an area of ongoing conflict between First Nations communities and the federal government.

## Veterans Affairs Canada

Through Veterans Affairs Canada (VAC) the federal government provides long-term institutional care for eligible veterans (VAC 2002). Care is provided to more than 550 veterans at Ste. Anne's Hospital outside of Montreal, the only remaining veterans' hospital administered by VAC. VAC also contracts with approximately 170 care facilities across Canada in order to ensure that priority access beds (PABs) are available to veterans. There are approximately 3,750 veterans residing in contract facilities offering PABs and another 4,500 veterans receiving long-term care in community care facilities across Canada. One study of institutionalized VAC clients notes that the average age upon admission is between 79 and 80 years (VAC 1997). And unlike other long-term care jurisdictions, VAC clients are 94 percent male, half of whom are married.

## Who Stays in Long-Term Care?

Only a very small percentage of the Canadian population resides in long-term care facilities (Havens 2002). In 1991, the figure was 1 percent of the total population. Residency in long-term care facilities is, not surprisingly, age-related. For those between the ages of 65 and 74 years, the percentage, while still small, nearly doubles to 1.8. A dramatic change is observed for those 85 years or older. Of this group, 33.9 percent are institutionalized in long-term care facilities. This undoubtedly reflects the increasing average age of admission, which has shifted over the past three decades from an average of 75 years in 1977 to an average of about 86 years (Pitters 2002).

The number of Canadians institutionalized is higher if we consider those individuals with disabilities (Havens 2002). Approximately 6 percent of the total Canadian population with disabilities and nearly half of all those 85 years or older with disabilities live in long-term care facilities (see Table 2.1).

The majority of long-term care residents are women. Between the ages of 65 and 74 the proportion of women to men is relatively equal (Pitters 2002); however, the proportion of women begins to outstrip men at about age 75 — perhaps reflecting women's longer life span or a lack of informal care. By the age of 85, women account for nearly two-thirds of the residents (see Table 2.2), prompting many to note that long-term care is not just a health issue but a women's issue.

Uncertainty around the impact of changing demographics is a key concern in long-term care policy and planning. The effects of the baby boom generation are of particular concern. Baby boomers will reach the key ages of 65 by 2011, 75 by 2021 and 85 by 2031 (Doupe et al. 2006). It is feared that the aging of baby boomers will increase the demands on the health care system, without a compensating increase in the workforce (who, given the current funding structure, pay for insured health services). According to Berta et al. (2006) the number of Canadians over the age of 65 will increase from 18.5 percent of the working-age population in 2001 to 33.6 percent in

**Table 2-1: Number and Percentage of People with Disabilities in Canada in 1991 by Age and Residence**

| Age Group | Living in Homes | | Living in Facilities | | Total |
|---|---|---|---|---|---|
| | # | % | # | % | |
| 0–14 | 389,350 | 100 | – | – | 389,350 |
| 15–34 | 675,055 | 98.4 | 11,205 | 1.6 | 686,255 |
| 35–54 | 992,830 | 97.8 | 22,215 | 2.2 | 1,015,055 |
| 55–64 | 629,245 | 97.5 | 15,895 | 2.5 | 645,135 |
| 65–74 | 698,830 | 95.4 | 33,885 | 4.6 | 732,715 |
| 75–84 | 424,800 | 83.6 | 83,035 | 16.4 | 507,835 |
| 85+ | 112,325 | 53.9 | 96,000 | 46.1 | 208,325 |
| Total | 3,922,435 | 93.7 | 262,235 | 6.3 | 4,184,670 |

*Source: Havens 2002*

**Table 2-2: Percent of Population in Long-term Care Facilities by Age and Sex, 1995**

| Age | Women (%) | Men (%) |
|---|---|---|
| 65–74 | 2 | 2 |
| 75–84 | 10 | 7 |
| 85+ | 38 | 24 |

*Source: Pitters 2002*

2026 and 41.0 percent in 2040. By the year 2051, almost 30 percent of the Canadian population will be over the age of 65.

Another way of looking at the likely expansion in demand for long-term care services is to consider that while the total Canadian population is expected to expand by 51 percent between 1991 and 2031, the population of those over 65 is predicted to increase by 182 percent (Havens 2002). This demand will not likely be distributed evenly across Canada. Not only will internal migration and immigration play a role in an unequal and changing geographic picture of long-term care, but at present, the elderly are not equally distributed across the country. In 1998, for instance 84 percent of seniors lived in four provinces (Ontario, Quebec, British Columbia and Alberta).

## Number and Type of Facilities

According to Statistics Canada's (2007c) survey, in 2005–2006 there were 2,086 residential care facilities catering to the elderly in Canada with a total of 206,170 beds (see Table 2.3). This represents a 13.7 percent increase in beds from the 2001–2002 survey. (Note that while Statistics Canada's Residential Care Facility survey is currently the only pan-Canadian data available, it should be interpreted with caution. In particular, the information collected by Statistics Canada is based on facilities' self-reporting. Further, not all facilities are included. In B.C., for instance, the survey does not include extended care units attached to hospitals; these tend to be better funded and staffed. As well, some retirement homes may be included in the data; these facilities tend to operate on a for-profit basis and typically cater to residents with lighter care needs. Group homes may also be included.)

The varied history of long-term care and mixed legislation has given rise to different types of facilities. Facility types are generally classified by ownership. Pitters (2002) has identified the following useful classifications:

- Proprietary (or for profit) — owned by an individual or corporation and run for profit.

**Table 2-3: Characteristics of Long-term Care in Canada**

| | |
|---|---|
| Facilities | 2,086 |
| Approved beds | 206,170 |
| Residents | 196,242 |
| Beds per facility | 95.5 |
| Full-time employees | 82,642 |
| Part-time employees | 76,090 |
| Paid hours | 335,127,707 |
| Salaries and wages ($) | 6,992,966,143 |
| Total expenses ($) | 10,852,242,676 |
| Total revenues ($) | 10,993,732,092 |
| Profit margin ($) | 141,489,416 |

*Source: Statistic Canada 2007c*

- Religious — owned and operated by a religious organization and not run for profit.
- Lay/charitable — owned and operated by a voluntary, non-governmental and non-religious body. Also not-for-profit.
- Municipal — owned and operated by a municipality on a not-for-profit basis.
- Regional — owned and operated by a regional health authority.
- Provincial/territorial — owned by a division of a provincial or territorial government.
- Federal — owned and operated by a department of the federal government.

For the most part, researchers tend to distinguish between profit and non-profit. Common as well are distinctions among government, religious and other not-for-profits and for-profit institutions. Using the latter distinctions, Berta et al. (2006) find that 25.2 percent of long-term care beds are in government-owned facilities, 10.2 percent in religious, 23.9 percent in not-for-profit and 40.7 percent in for-profit facilities. For a detailed regional breakdown see Table 2.4.

Clearly, there is considerable regional variation. In the Atlantic provinces, for-profits dominate, accounting for 40 percent of long-term care beds. In contrast, in Alberta, the Prairies and Ontario, government ownership prevails, with over 40 percent in each region. The situation is more or less evenly split between for-profits and not-for-profits in British Columbia, with a minimal percentage of government (10 percent) and religious (8 percent) beds.

Recalling the earlier caveats around long-term care statistics, a considerably different picture emerges if ownership patterns for long-term care

**Table 2-4: Ownership Type by Region, 2001**

| Region | Ownership | % |
|---|---|---|
| Atlantic | For-profit | 40 |
| | Government | 22 |
| | Not-for-profit | 28 |
| | Religious | 10 |
| Ontario | For-profit | 17 |
| | Government | 46 |
| | Not-for-profit | 18 |
| | Religious | 19 |
| Prairies | For-profit | 17 |
| | Government | 46 |
| | Not-for-profit | 18 |
| | Religious | 19 |
| Alberta | For-profit | 21 |
| | Government | 41 |
| | Not-for-profit | 22 |
| | Religious | 16 |
| British Columbia | For-profit | 38 |
| | Government | 10 |
| | Not-for-profit | 44 |
| | Religious | 8 |

*Source: Berta et al. 2006*

facilities (rather than beds) is examined and especially if government and religious facilities are included in the not-for-profit category. Consider the breakdown in Table 2.5, provided by the Ontario Health Coalition.

When analyzing data by beds versus facilities, differences may be partially explained by the fact that the number of beds varies by institutional type. In other words, some institutional types tend to be bigger than others. As Berta et al. (2006: 180) observe:

> Government owned facilities are significantly larger than For-Profit and Not-for-Profit facilities, with a mean facility size of 77 LTC beds. Facilities owned by Religious organizations are significantly larger than For-Profits and Not-for-Profits, with a mean size of 74 beds compared to 50 and 30 beds respectively. Lay Not-for Profits operate the smallest facilities with an average facility size of 30 LTC beds.

### Table 2-5: Ownership Type by Selected Provinces

| Province | Public/Not-for-profit (%) | Private for-profit (%) |
|---|---|---|
| British Columbia | 68.3 | 31.7 |
| Saskatchewan | 96.2 | 5.8 |
| Manitoba | 84.0 | 15.0 |
| Ontario | 48.4 | 51.6 |
| New Brunswick | 100.0 | 0 |
| Nova Scotia | 72.0 | 28.0 |

*Source: OHC 2002*

## Who Pays for Long-Term Care?

To the degree that funding for long-term care comes from the federal government, it arrives through a block transfer to provinces and territories. There is no targeted federal funding for long-term care.

Provinces are responsible for system design, funding allocation, policy development and regulatory compliance. Provinces cost-share long-term care with residents through the application of a set — often income-dependent — monthly accommodation rate (see Table 2.6). In some provinces, this rate varies with the type of room (e.g., one pays more for private accommodation). In Quebec, for instance, the 2008 maximum rate for a bed in a room with three or more other beds is $988.50. This rate increases to $1,329.00 for a "semi-private" room and $1,590.90 for a private room (RAMQ 2008).

## Entry to Long-Term Care

Individuals generally access long-term care through a single entry point system in order to ensure their needs are correctly assessed and they are appropriately placed within the continuum of care. These entry points are often established and coordinated by regional health authorities or other local bodies.

In Quebec, for instance, someone finding it difficult to support themselves would approach (or have a caregiver approach) their local "health and social service centre" (CSSS). There a "multiclientele tool" — which is used across the province — would help determine the level of care required and whether or not it can be met by home care, "intermediate resources" or residential and long-term care centres (RLTCCs in Quebec). This assessment tool, as with most others, inquires into one's state of health, one's ability to conduct daily activities and one's level of social support. If the individual is able to remain at home with the addition of psychosocial services (often provided by social workers) and/or home support services such as meals and housekeeping (often provided by volunteer agencies), some form of home care is organized. If the level of care required is greater than this, the individuals will likely be directed to an intermediate form of housing. If 24-hour nursing care is *not* required then this might be some form of assisted living or supportive housing. This type of housing is not the focus of this chapter and would appear to vary widely across the country in terms of ownership, fee structure, design and integration into local health networks. If, on the other hand, 24-hour nursing care *is* required, then the individual will enter long-term residential care, or more likely be put on a wait list.

## Health Needs and Care Provision

The typical long-term care resident has some form of cognitive impairment, has difficulty moving independently, is incontinent, suffers from chronic (often multiple) diseases and may have lost a spouse or partner. As noted above, the typical long-term care resident is an elderly women with an average age of 85.

A study by PricewaterhouseCoopers (2001) provides a useful indication of the types of impairments faced by long-term care residents. It examines data from a number of Canadian provinces, U.S. states and Nordic countries. The most common diagnoses found were dementia and/or Alzheimer's, and with few exceptions over half the residents in the various sites studied were diagnosed with such. Cognitive impairment and a fair to high degree

**Table 2-6: Basic Accommodation Rates of Provinces, as of 2007**

| Province | Minimum Monthly Accommodation Rates | Maximum Monthly Accommodation Rates |
|---|---|---|
| British Columbia | $882 | $2118 |
| Alberta | $1354 | $1650 |
| Saskatchewan | $956 | $1815 |
| Manitoba | $903 | $2120 |
| Ontario | $1578 | $2125 |
| Quebec | $988 | $1590 |
| Newfoundland & Labrador | $2800 | |
| New Brunswick | $2129 | |
| Nova Scotia | $2403 | |
| Prince Edward Island | $1977 | $3011 |

*Source: Ministry Websites*

of difficulty with the activities of daily living were found in nearly half of all residents. Depression was also relatively common, found in around 10 to 30 percent of residents. Common physical impairments were arthritis, diabetes, stroke and congestive heart failure.

While such broad-based inter-provincial and international comparisons provide an idea of the "typical" long-term care resident, there are also important differences that can only be assessed by inquiring into the distribution of resident health status among specific long-term care institutions and ownership types. Berta et al. (2006), for instance, find that residents requiring more complex care predominantly reside in government-owned facilities, though there is considerable variability across the country. Table 2.7 illustrates the way the most intense level of care (Type 3 Care: specifying a minimum requirement of 2.5 hours of direct care and the 24-hour avail-

**Table 2-7: Care Levels and Amount by Region and Ownership Type, 2001**

| Region | Ownership | % of 'Beds' with Type 3 Care | Total Hours of Direct Care | RN+RNA Care Hours |
|---|---|---|---|---|
| | For-profit | 4 | 1.98 | 0.91 |
| | Government | 31 | 8.32 | 2.57 |
| | Not for profit | 42 | 5.91 | 1.84 |
| Atlantic | Religious | 23 | 3.27 | 2.18 |
| | For profit | 46 | 2.41 | 0.66 |
| | Government | 39 | 4.26 | 1.15 |
| | Not for profit | 8 | 5.79 | 1.13 |
| Ontario | Religious | 7 | 3.90 | 0.8 |
| | For profit | 19 | 2.69 | 1.24 |
| | Government | 53 | 4.22 | 1.68 |
| | Not for profit | 10 | 5.56 | 1.49 |
| Prairies | Religious | 18 | 3.47 | 1.96 |
| | For profit | 9 | 4.44 | 1.59 |
| | Government | 65 | 5.20 | 3.30 |
| | Not for profit | 14 | 5.68 | 1.87 |
| Alberta | Religious | 12 | 4.84 | 2.32 |
| | For profit | 32 | 4.12 | 1.02 |
| | Government | 14 | 5.13 | 1.60 |
| | Not for profit | 45 | 6.62 | 1.20 |
| B.C. | Religious | 9 | 4.30 | 1.25 |

*Source: Compiled from Berta et al. 2006.*

ability of nursing care) distributes among region and ownership type.

As Berta et al. (2006) suggest, there are a number of reasons to assume a relationship between both level of care and amount of direct care provided (measured in terms of hours), and there is also reason to assume facility ownership type might influence the levels of care provided. Table 2.7 also provides a description of the average amount of care provided in various institutions. Their analysis suggests that not-for-profit lay organizations offer the highest levels of direct care at an average of 5.96 hours a day. This is compared to 5.22 hours for government, 3.96 hours for religious and 2.71 hours for for-profit institutions. Furthermore, it would seem that care is provided by different workers, depending on the type of institution. Government-run facilities provide the highest level of professional nursing care, whereas in not-for-profit facilities the highest proportion of direct care is provided by aides or workers other than registered nurses or registered nursing assistants.

## Long-Term Care in Selected Provinces

### Nova Scotia

There are three types of long-term continuing care homes in Nova Scotia operating under the jurisdiction of the Department of Health. These are: nursing homes, residential care facilities and community-based options (Department of Health 2007). While this overview focuses on nursing homes, the basic features of the three types of residences are described below.

*Community-based options* (CBOs) provide care for seniors for whom home care is no longer appropriate and nursing home care is not required. CBOs are small home-like supportive environments that typically serve a maximum of three individuals. They provide personal care by workers available on site 24 hours a day. Such care may include help with bathing and dressing, administration of medication, meal service as well as reminders about daily routines. Residents have a private bedroom and share common areas (dining room, bathroom and outdoor space). There are currently 28 CBOs in Nova Scotia, though most are in the Sydney and Halifax areas. They are privately owned and operated.

*Residential care facilities* (RCFs) provide an intermediate level of care for people who need supervision and non-nursing personal care. RCFs may operate either under the jurisdiction of the Department of Health or the Department of Community Services. RCFs under the Department of Health provide care mainly to the elderly and provide personal care that may include help with bathing and dressing, meals, administration of medication and reminders about daily routines. RCFs have a care worker available 24 hours a day. RCFs are mostly owned and operated by private individuals or

| Nova Scotia LTC in Numbers | |
| --- | --- |
| Nursing homes | 71 |
| Beds | 5835 |
| Non-profit homes | 29 |
| For-profit homes | 21 |
| Residential care facilities | 35 |
| Community-based options | 28 |
| | |
| Gender in nursing homes | 71% women |
| 85 years and older | 43% |
| Accommodation cost | $2265/month |

organizations. Residents either have a private bedroom or share with one other person. There are currently 35 RCFs in Nova Scotia, ranging from 6 beds to 85 beds each.

*Nursing homes* — also referred to as homes for the aged — are facilities provided for people who need high levels of nursing care. Nursing homes operate under the jurisdiction of the Department of Health and serve primarily seniors, although there are some young adult residents and one children's unit in the province. There are 71 nursing homes in Nova Scotia with a total of 5,835 beds. Facilities range in size from 5 to 538 beds and are of mixed ownership. Twenty-two are municipally owned, 21 are private for-profit and 7 are hospital-based.

### Regulation of Long-Term Care in Nova Scotia

Long-term care in Nova Scotia is administered through the Nova Scotia Department of Health's Continuing Care Branch. In addition to long-term care, the Continuing Care Branch administers home care and the adult protection services (i.e., protection for vulnerable adults). All long-term care facilities fall under the jurisdiction of the *Homes for Special Care Act*.

### Who Pays and How Much?

Long-term care is paid for jointly by the provincial government and by long-term care residents (Department of Health 2007).

In Nova Scotia the provincial government covers the health care costs for each resident. These costs may be related to the salaries, benefits and operational costs of nursing and personal care; social work services; recreation therapy; and physical, occupational and other therapies. These costs will only be covered for residents who enter long-term care homes that participate in the provincial single entry access system.

Residents are expected to pay the accommodation charges, which include salaries, benefits and operational costs of maintenance, dietary services, housekeeping, management and administration departments, capital and return on investment. This charge is collected by the long-term care facility. Accommodation costs effective November 1, 2007, were $79.00 per day for nursing homes, $50.50 for RCFs and $46.50 for CBOs (Department of Health 2007).

Reduced accommodation charges are available, though a yearly needs assessment is required. As of January 2005, this assessment no longer includes the resident's financial assets in order to prevent residents from drawing down their assets to pay for accommodation costs. This assessment also accounts for spouses who remain at home, allowing them to retain 50 percent of the joint family income and control over all assets.

Personal expenses must be paid by the resident (e.g., clothing, eyeglasses, hearing aids, dental services, funerals, pharmacare co-payment and transportation). However, transportation for dialysis or inter-facility transfers is paid by the province. There is also a specialized equipment loan program available for residents in long-term care. This program is administered by the Red Cross. Depending on income, residents may be required to pay a fee.

### Who Stays in Long-Term Care?

Admission to the three types of long-term care facilities in Nova Scotia is centralized through the Single Entry Access System of the Continuing Care Branch. They assess the level of care required and determine the most appropriate type of institution.

RCFs and CBOs are intended for residents with similar health capacities (Department of Health 2007). A typical RCF or CBO resident is someone who has care needs that cannot be safely provided at home. While they generally have decreased physical and/or mental abilities, they are mobile (with or without the assistance of canes, wheelchairs, walkers) and they do *not* require more than 1.5 hours a day of supervision or personal care. They also do not require the services of an on-site registered nurse. CBO residents also do not typically require night-time care. RCF and CBO residents commonly suffer from chronic diseases such as arthritis and hypertension. Yet in case of emergency they must be able to vacate the premises unassisted.

Women comprise the majority (71 percent) of nursing home residents (CIHI 2006). While 5 percent of residents are under the age of 65, most (43 percent) are 85 years old or more, twenty percent of residents are between the ages of 75 and 84. Between the ages of 75· and 84 the proportion of women to men is roughly 2 to 1. This increases to a ratio of more than 3 to 1 for residents over 85 years of age (see Table 2.8).

As is to be expected, nursing home residents suffer from more aggravated

**Table 2-8: Age and Sex Distribution as Percentage of Total Resident Population**

| Age Group | Female | Male | All |
|---|---|---|---|
| Younger than 65 | 2% | 3% | 5% |
| 65 to 74 | 6% | 3% | 9% |
| 75 to 84 | 20% | 11% | 31% |
| 85 and older | 43% | 12% | 55% |
| All Ages | 71% | 29% | 100% |

*Source: CIHI 2006*

and complex health conditions (CIHI 2006). The most common diagnoses were Alzheimer's and dementia (64 percent of residents). Sixty percent showed moderate to severe cognitive impairment, 44 percent showed limited or no social engagement and 18 percent showed signs of depression. Nearly one third (31 percent) experienced daily unrelieved pain, with an additional 5 percent experiencing severe daily pain. The most common physical conditions experienced by residents were hypertension (45 percent), arthritis (31 percent) and diabetes (26 percent).

## Ontario

Residential continuing care in Ontario is delivered through three mechanisms: retirement homes, supportive housing and long-term care facilities (MOHLTC 2008). These forms of housing are distinguished principally by level of care, though cost, ownership structure and governing legislation are also key points of distinction. While this overview focuses on long-term care facilities, the basic features of the three types of residences are described below.

*Retirement homes* — also referred to as retirement residences, care homes, assisted living and rest homes — are intended for individuals or couples requiring a minimum level of support (e.g., light housekeeping, social activities, meals, low levels of personal care and, depending on the institution, availability of staff on a 24-hours basis). These homes are largely run by private, for-profit corporations (though there are a small number of non-profits), and cost can vary from $1500 per month for a private room to $5000. While some municipalities may have "care home" by-laws, these institutions are not governed by special legislation and thus fall under the *Tenant Protection Act*. Unlike long-term care institutions, individuals apply directly to the provider for admittance.

*Supportive housing* — also known as non-profit housing, social housing, senior's housing — is intended for those who require a greater amount of care, though *not* 24-hour nursing or specialized care. Supportive housing provides daily personal care, meal preparation and homemaking support,

| Ontario LTC in Numbers | |
|---|---|
| Total beds in 2004 | 70,100 |
| Total LTC homes | 577 |
| For-profit homes | 343 |
| Non-profit homes | 68 |
| Municipal homes | 102 |
| Charitable homes | 64 |
| Per diems (per resident) | $51.88–69.88 in 2008 |
| Accommodation cost | $1578 to $2125 per month in 2008 |
| Average age | 83 |
| Sex | 76.6% women |
| Care (RN, RPN, aide) | 2.04 hrs |

as well as the 24-hour availability of a personal support worker. While building management varies, the provision of services is managed by non-profit corporations and covered by the Ontario Ministry of Health and Long-term Care (MOHLTC). Costs range from $699 to $1200 per month and rent subsidies are available in some locations. Residence buildings within supportive housing are governed by the *Tenant Protection Act*, while the *Long-Term Care Homes Act* governs service provision. Individuals apply directly to the provider for admittance.

*Long-term care homes* — also referred to as nursing homes or homes for the aged — are intended for those who require specialized daily personal care and the availability of 24-hour nursing care and/or supervision. The majority of long-term care homes in Ontario are owned by private, for-profit corporations, although there are a number owned and operated by non-profit corporations and municipal governments. While the MOHLTC provides funding, resident co-payment is required, with rates set by the ministry according to the type of room. Long-term care facilities are governed by the *Long-Term Care Homes Act* and admission is processed through one of the 14 Community Care Access Centres (CCACs) in Ontario.

### Number of Facilities and Ownership Type

The most recently available figures show that in 2004 there were 70,850 long-term care beds in Ontario, up from 57,000 beds in 2000 (Smith 2004). More than half of these beds (38,057) are in for-profit homes, compared to 16,654 beds in municipal homes, 6,588 beds in non-profit homes and 8,841 beds in charitable homes. This represents the highest proportion of private sector involvement in the country (OHC 2002).

### Regulation of Long-term Care in Ontario

Until the mid-1960s two statutes governed long-term care facilities in Ontario: the *Homes for the Aged and Rest Homes Act* (1949) and the *Charitable Institutions Act* (1951). Homes for the aged were operated by municipalities, and charitable homes were operated by charities. Both were non-profit enterprises. There were also number of private for-profit nursing homes that went unregulated until the introduction of the *Nursing Homes Act* in 1966.

In 1994, Bill101 and Bill 173, *The Long-Term Care Act,* was passed to bring nursing homes, homes for the aged and charitable homes under the purview of one ministry. This move towards consolidation was furthered by the passing of Bill 140, *An Act Respecting Long-term Care Homes,* in June 2007. The new Act came on the heels of a number of "scandals" and poor evaluations of long-term care facilities in Ontario (McKay 2003a; PWC 2001). Not surprisingly, the Act was touted as strengthening enforcement and improving care and accountability. Among other things, the Act stipulated the following:

- yearly unannounced facility inspections with reports made publicly available in LTC facilities and online;
- whistle-blowing protections for persons, including staff, residents and volunteers, who report abuse or neglect;
- a detailed "least restraint policy" limiting the use of restraints and including appropriate safeguards;
- an enhanced and more clearly enforceable Residents' Bill of Rights; and
- strengthened requirements related to the development of an integrated, interdisciplinary plan of care for every resident.

Regulation of long-term care facilities is also provided through Residents' and Family Councils, autonomous bodies that act as advocates for seniors in homes, advising residents of their rights, monitoring facility operations, reviewing inspection reports and financial statements, and filing complaints. As of 2004, there were 178 Residents' Councils and 154 Family Councils within long-term care facilities (Smith 2004). The *Long-Term Care Act* mandates the establishment of Residents' Councils in each home and strongly encourages the creation of Family Councils.

Finally, there is a toll-free ACTION line (1-866-434-0144) available for residents and home care clients to voice complaints, concerns and questions. The 2007 Act expanded this service to include family members.

### Who Pays and How Much?

As noted, while the MOHLTC provides funding for long-term care institutions, residents are required to make a "co-payment" dependent on the type of room (MOHLTC 2008). As of November 2008 room rates were $1578.02 per month for basic accommodations (e.g., a room shared among four people), $1821.35 for semi-private and $2125.52 for private accommodations. Government subsidies are available for basic accommodation only. As 60 percent of available beds are reserved for those who can pay the additional daily fee for "preferred" accommodation, these may remain empty while there are wait lists for "basic" accommodation (Smith 2004).

### How is Long-Term Care Funding Determined?

In 1993, the Ministry of Health set out a new needs-based funding system for long-term care facilities (OHC 2002). Residents are assessed annually by the ministry and categorized according to the Albert Classification System, which measures eight indicators of care requirements: eating, toileting, transferring, dressing, potential for injury to self or others, ineffective coping, urinary continence and bowel continence. This information is then aggregated to provide a sense of the total care requirements for each facility or what is called a Case Mix Measure. By averaging the Case Mix Measure for all facilities, a Case Mix Index is produced, which enables the ministry to determine baseline funding levels. The funds allocated to each facility depend on where it falls in relation to this average.

At the time of writing, the Ontario Ministry of Health and Long-Term Care is moving towards the use of the Resident Assessment Instrument Minimum Data Set or RAI-MDS 2.0. The RAI-MDS 2.0 was developed by InterRAI, a global team of researchers and clinicians. It is a care planning tool designed to be used in long-term care facilities where skilled nursing services are employed (e.g., both nursing homes and chronic care hospitals). In addition to care planning, it supports quality indicator reporting, outcome measures and case mix classification through its Resource Utilization Groupings (RUGs). RUGs are often used in resource allocation planning. The RAI-MDS 2.0 is mandated for use across the United States, is increasingly being used in Europe and is slowly becoming the standard assessment tool in Canada. As of 2007, 35 percent of Ontario's long-term care facilities have adopted the RAI-MDS 2.0, while 65 percent of facilities still employ the Alberta Classification System (Sharkey 2008).

Long-term care funding in Ontario is allocated through the following four envelopes: 1) nursing care and personal care; 2) program and support services; 3) raw food; and 4) accommodation costs (facility costs, administration, housekeeping, building and operational maintenance, and dietary and laundry services). The amount allocated for nursing and personal support is based on the Case Mix Index described above. The amounts for programming and support as well as for accommodation are set by the province and are the same for every institution. With the exception of accommodation — which is paid by the resident — all unused funds must be returned to the province. Thus accommodation is the only envelope from which for-profit facilities may extract capital.

Table 2.9 illustrates that in 2001 the total per diem rate amounted to $102 for an "average" long-term care resident — or $57.62 if we do not include the amount paid by the resident herself. As McKay (2003a) observes, public funds for long-term care residents are considerably less than the $140 per diem spent on inmates in jails and detention centres.

### Who Stays in Long-Term Care?

Women comprise the majority (76.6 percent) of long-term care residents in Ontario (PWC 2001). The average age of long-term care residents is 83 years (Sharkey 2008).

Long-term care residents cope with a complex mix of age-related physical diseases and cognitive challenges (PWC 2001). Several measures assessing levels of impairment find that almost half of long-term care residents in Ontario (44.8 percent) show high levels of cognitive impairment, and 47.9 percent show high impairment when it comes to independence in activities of daily living. More specifically, over half of Ontario residents (53 percent) have been diagnosed with some form of dementia (including Alzheimer's). When assessed with a depression rating scale, 30.5 percent of residents indicate the presence of minor or major depression. Physically, 70 percent of residents suffer from incontinence, 19 percent from diabetes, 22 percent from stroke, 30 percent from arthritis, and 11 percent have congestive heart failure.

It is well known, though perhaps less well documented, that residents in long-term care facilities are entering older and requiring increasingly more care (OHC 2008). According to the Ontario Association of Non-Profit Homes and Services for Seniors (in OHC 2002), for instance, care requirements of residents increased an average of 13.7 percent between 1993 and 2001. The greatest increase — of 30.8 percent — was seen in charitable homes for the aged, twice that of municipal homes (15 percent). Nursing homes evidenced the smallest increase in acuity levels: 9.9 percent.

### Table 2-9: Breakdown of Per Diem Rates per Resident, as of October 1, 2001

| Envelope | Amount |
|---|---|
| Nursing and personal care (average CMI) | $52.38 |
| Programming and support services | $5.24 |
| Accommodation<br>(Including the "raw food" amount of $4.49 per day)* | $44.70 |
| Total | $102.32 |

*Starting in 2004, raw food began to be treated as a separate envelope.

*Source: OHC 2002*

In sum, according to the PriceWaterhouseCoopers (2001) survey, Ontario long-term care residents are among the oldest, have one of the highest rates of mental impairment and are the most depressed.

## Manitoba

Residential continuing care in Manitoba is delivered in the following three forms: assisted living, supportive housing and personal care homes (Manitoba Health 2007b).While this chapter focuses on long-term care facilities (called personal care homes or PCHs), the basic features of the three types of residences are discussed below.

*Assisted living* combines independent apartment living with purchased services such as housekeeping, meals and laundry. Individuals must apply and contract directly with the landlord. Some sites provide supervision and assistance and individuals have access to provincial or local programs — such as home care — which are currently being deepened through Manitoba Health's Aging in Place strategy.

*Supportive housing* provides intermediate personal care to individuals requiring 24-hour support and supervision. Supportive housing targets mainly seniors and houses individuals in group community settings. While the province funds the health care component, the individuals pay for rent and any additional support services (e.g., housekeeping, meals, laundry). Some locations may have rental assistance but the majority do not. Within the Winnipeg Regional Health Authority (WRHA), for instance, only 20 of the 272 spaces offer rent geared to income (WRHA 2007).

It is worth noting that supportive housing and assisted living are sometimes found in combination. One such site is the Riverside Lions Seniors Residences in St. Vital, a suburban section of Winnipeg (WHHI 2007). This complex is a fully accessible five-storey, 75-unit apartment building that is

| Manitoba LTC in Numbers | |
| --- | --- |
| Beds (2006) | 9822 |
| Occupancy rate | 96% |
| Institutions | 122 |
| Not-for-profit | 103 |
| For-profit | 19 |
| Average age | 83 |
| Per diem (resident charge) | $28.80 to $67.60 |
| Sex ratio: | |
| 75 to 84 years | 2:1 (women: men) |
| 85 + years | 3:1 (women: men) |

to be linked with another independent living seniors' building nearby. The completed $2-million-dollar project will have 27 one-bedroom units offering assisted living and 48 supportive housing studio units for seniors with early-stage dementia/Alzheimer's.

*Personal care homes* (PCHs) are facility-based settings providing 24-hour professional nursing services to those who can no longer manage to live independently at home with family and/or home care support. Residents pay a daily, income-based rate set by Manitoba Health. The province also funds the health care component. According to Manitoba Health (2007b), PCHs offer the following services:

- meals (including meals for special diets);
- assistance with daily living activities like bathing, getting dressed and using the bathroom;
- necessary nursing care;
- routine medical and surgical supplies;
- prescription drugs eligible under Manitoba's Personal Care Home Program;
- physiotherapy and occupational therapy, if the facility is approved to provide these services; and
- routine laundry and linen services.

### Number of Facilities and Ownership Type

In June 2004 there were 122 personal care homes (PCHs) in Manitoba with a total of 9,586 beds (Doupe et al. 2006). By 2006 the number of beds had increased to 9,822 (Manitoba Health 2007a).

PCHs are not evenly distributed across the province. The largest proportion of PCHs (31.1 percent) was located in the district covered by the Winnipeg Regional Health Authority (Doupe et al. 2006; WRHA 2007). Since these institutions tend to be bigger, over half (57.6 percent) of the total PCH beds in the province are concentrated in the WRHA (see Table 2.10).

PCHs in Manitoba are classified as proprietary (for-profit) and non-proprietary (not-for-profit). In 2004, 84 percent or 103 PCHs were non-proprietary (Doupe et al. 2006) and 16 percent were run for profit. PCH facilities in Manitoba are further classified as freestanding or juxtaposed to another health care facility. All proprietary facilities are freestanding. In contrast, 64 non-proprietary facilities are freestanding (or 52.5 percent of the PCHs in Manitoba) compared to 39 juxtaposed PCHs (or 32 percent of the provincial total).

Given the concentration of beds in Winnipeg, the WRHA (2007) data are worth examining more closely. As of 2007, there were 39 PCHs in Winnipeg, for a total of 5,697 PCH beds (up by almost 200 beds from 2004). Of these, 3,555 beds were within the 25 non-proprietary PCHs. The 14 proprietary

**Table 2-10: Number and Percent of PCH Facilities and Beds in Manitoba, by Regional Health Authority (RHA)**

| RHA | PCHs | Beds |
|---|---|---|
| Assiniboine | 27 (22.1%) | 909 (9.5%) |
| Brandon | 5 (4.1%) | 597 (6.2%) |
| Central | 15 (12.3%) | 831 (8.7%) |
| Interlake | 11 (9%) | 552 (5.8%) |
| Norman | 3 (2.5%) | 126 (1.3%) |
| North Eastman | 5 (4.1%) | 190 (2%) |
| Parkland | 11 (9%) | 544 (5.7%) |
| South Eastman | 7 (5.7%) | 334 (3.5%) |
| Non-Winnipeg Total | 84 (68.9%) | 4,083 (42.6%) |
| Winnipeg | 38 (31.1%) | 5,503 (57.4%) |
| Manitoba Total | 122 (100%) | 9,586 (100%) |

Source: Doupe et al. 2006

PCHs have 2,142 beds. Not all beds are for the elderly. The WRHA reports that of the 5,697 beds, there are

- 4,977 general personal beds;
- 352 behavioural special needs beds;
- 36 beds for young disabled adults;
- 20 beds for deaf or hearing impaired individuals;
- 9 behavioural treatment beds;
- 249 interim Personal Care Home beds; and
- 34 respite beds.

### Recent Policy Developments

Admission to PCHs falls under the Manitoba Home Care Program. This program was established in 1974 as the first province-wide, coordinated, continuing care program in Canada. Manitoba Health administered the program until 1997, when regional health authorities assumed control for the majority of functions, including assessment and admissions to PCHs.

In January 2006 Manitoba Health launched a new long-term care strategy for seniors, called Aging in Place (Manitoba Health 2006). This program is intended to address the fact that Manitoba has the highest rate of PCH placements in the country (126 beds per 1000 over the age of 75). High PCH placement is perceived to be a significant problem. The aim of the strategy is therefore to maximize community living options. Nevertheless, Aging in Place incorporates plans to improve PCH environments by moving

**Table 2-11: Number and Percent of PCHs in Manitoba by Ownership Type**

| RHA | Total # of PCHs | Non-Proprietary PCHs | Proprietary PCHs |
|---|---|---|---|
| Assiniboine | 27 | 27 (60%) | 0 |
| Brandon | 5 | 3 (60%) | 2 (40%) |
| Central | 15 | 15 (100%) | 0 |
| Interlake | 11 | 9 (81.8%) | 2 (18.2%) |
| Norman | 3 | 3 (100%) | 0 |
| North Eastman | 5 | 5 (100%) | 0 |
| Parkland | 11 | 11 (100%) | 0 |
| South Eastman | 7 | 6 (85.5%) | 1 (14%) |
| Non-Winnipeg | 84 | 79 (94%) | 5 (6%) |
| Winnipeg | 38 | 24 (63.2%) | 14 (36.8%) |
| Manitoba | 122 (100%) | 103 (84.4%) | 19 (15.6%) |

Source: Doupe et al. 2006

towards single-bed accommodations rather than shared accommodations. For instance, in Winnipeg, approximately 70 percent of PCH beds are in single rooms. The Aging in Place goal is to raise this to 97 percent within five years. In keeping with the continuing care model, Aging in Place provides $98 million for, among other things: supportive housing and supports for seniors in group living.

### Who Pays and How Much?

The costs of staying at a PCH are shared by the province and the resident (Manitoba Health 2007b). Manitoba Health pays the majority of the cost through regional health authorities. The individual pays an income-based "residential charge" that is set annually. In 2007, residential charges ranged from $28.80 per day to a maximum of $67.60 per day. As with other provinces, the residential charge structure is intended to ensure that residents retain a certain amount of disposable income for personal expenses. In 2007 the allowed amount was a minimum $254 per month or $3,048 per year for those paying the minimum residential charge. Spousal "allowances" are also calculated and, for a resident paying the minimum, can range from $13,356 to $27,925.

### Who Stays in Long-Term Care?

In 2000, Manitoba had the highest rate of PCH placement in the country at 126 beds per 1000 people over the age of 75. Most residents (93 percent) entering PCHs come from home care (Roos et al. 2001). The average resident is 83 years old, female and resides in a PCH for 2.8 years (Manitoba Health 2007a).

In a study of PCH residents from 1999 to 2003, Doupe et al. (2006) found that half of all residents admitted during this five-year period were 85 years or older. About one-third (36.2 percent) were between the ages of 75 and 84, while only 9.9 percent of admissions were for people between 65 and 74. Younger people were admitted, though they comprised only 3.9 percent of all admissions.

As in other provinces, residents of long-term care tend to be elderly women (Doupe et al. 2006). While the sex distribution is relatively equal up to the age of 74, beyond this the proportion of women begins to outstrip men. Residents between 75 and 84 years of age are twice as likely to be women and residents 85 years or older are more than three times as likely to be women (Doupe et al. 2006). Similarly, there is a significant sex difference in marital status. While 26 percent of both men and women younger than 75 are married, nearly half (40.2 percent) of men 75 years or older are married. This compares to only 11.5 percent of women 75 years or older. This means that women are less likely to have a spouse to provide informal care — one of the taken-for-granted assumptions of many home care programs.

The health care needs of residents are not particularly surprising. The majority (65.3 percent) of PCH residents had been diagnosed with dementia (Doupe et al. 2006). And many, if not most, residents (70 percent) suffered from two or more chronic diseases. The most common of these was arthritis (28 percent), followed by diabetes (17 percent), stroke (16 percent) and congestive heart failure (13 percent)(PWC 2001).

## British Columbia

In British Columbia long-term care is administered through the Community Care Facilities Branch (CCFB) of the provincial government, which provides residential elderly care through assisted living and residential care facilities (Ministry of Health 2007b). Although this chapter focuses on residential care facilities (RCFs), both types of housing services are described below.

*Assisted living residences* — also referred to as supportive housing — provide housing and care to seniors and people with disabilities who can direct their own care and do not require the availability of 24-hour nursing care. Assisted living residences combine hospitality services such as laundry and housekeeping with personal assistance, such as help with eating, the monitoring of medications and mobility assistance. Assisted living is distinguished from residential facility care by the number of "prescribed services" provided. Only one or two prescribed services are provided. Residents are therefore required to self-direct most of their care. Residents of publicly funded assisted living residences pay a monthly charge based on their after-tax income.

*Residential facility care (RCFs)* forms part of what the CCFB refers more generally to as *licensed community care facilities*. Licensed community care facilities include both child day care facilities (e.g., preschool, day care) and residential care facilities (RCFs) for adults. The term "residential care facility" does not refer only to senior care, but to group homes for disabled individuals and drug and alcohol rehabilitation facilities. RCFs are typically sites where care is provided to three or more individuals. Residents of RCFs pay a per diem amount based on their after-tax income. RCFs are distinguished from assisted living because they provide three or more prescribed services, which may include:

- regular assistance with daily activities (e.g., mobility, eating, dressing, grooming, bathing and personal hygiene);
- monitoring of food intake or therapeutic diets;
- administering and monitoring of medication;
- distribution of medication;
- maintenance or management of residents' cash and valuables;
- structured behaviour management and intervention; and
- psychosocial and physical rehabilitative therapy.

In addition to RCFs, B.C. also has *family care homes*, which are single family residences that provide supportive accommodation for up to two clients. Family care homes may serve as an alternative to staying at an RCF. While they are found across the province, family care homes are more prevalent in rural settings.

As well, B.C. has *group homes*, which are private residences geared primarily towards adults with disabilities. Group homes are similar but larger than Abbeyfield housing, a type of shared supportive housing based on a model developed in Great Britain. An Abbeyfield house resembles a large house where residents have a private room, sometimes a private bathroom, but share other living spaces. Meals, cleaning support and other non-nursing forms of assistance are provided by a housekeeper. Abbeyfield-type housing is becoming common in British Columbia.

| British Columbia LTC in Numbers | |
|---|---|
| Ownership Type | Percent of Beds |
| For-profit | 38% |
| Not-for-profit | 44% |
| Government | 10% |
| Religious | 8% |
| Monthly cost | $882 to $2118 |

### Number of Facilities and Ownership Type

British Columbia has the lowest long-term care bed capacity in the country (Berta et al. 2006). In 2001 there were 3.6 beds for every 100 individuals over the age of 65. This proportion has decreased slightly from 1996, when it was at 3.8. The majority of residential care beds are located in either non-profit (44 percent) or for-profit (38 percent) facilities. In B.C., government-run facilities comprise only 10 percent of the long-term care beds. This is similar to religious facilities, which have 8 percent of the provincial beds.

### Regulation of Long-Term Care Facilities

Long-term care is administered through the Community Care Facilities Branch (CCFB) of the B.C. Ministry of Health. The CCFB is responsible for the development and implementation of legislation, policy and guidelines to protect the health and safety of people being cared for in long-term care facilities.

Long-term care facilities are regulated by the *Community Care and Assisted Living Act* (Ministry of Health 2007a). This act was brought into force on May 14, 2004, replacing the *Community Care Facilities Act*. The new Act enumerates the type of prescribed services that may be provided. As noted above, the number of prescribed services differentiates a licensed community care facility from an assisted living residence. The Act also requires operators of assisted living residences to register with the provincial Office of the Assisted Living Registrar. The Registrar maintains a registry of assisted living residences and investigates health and safety concerns.

The Act brings under its purview public extended care facilities, which have provided 24/7 professional nursing care for seniors and people with disabilities. These institutions used to operate under the 1996 *Hospital Act*, the same legislation as public acute care hospitals. Transferring these facilities to the new Act is intended to ensure that they are consistent with licensed residential care facilities, which provide similar services.

### Who Pays for Long-Term Care?

The province shares the cost of long-term care through accommodation charges, which are generally income adjusted. In 2007, the RCF per diem rate ranged from a minimum of $29.40 to a maximum of $70.60. Family care homes are operated under the same fixed cost structure, whereas group home rental rates are set by the landlord. The province also sets rates for residents of assisted living. These rates are based on 70 percent of the resident's after-tax income.

### Senior Demographics and Facility Residency

B.C. has one of the most rapidly aging populations in Canada (Ministry of Health 2004). Between 1991 and 2001, the median age in B.C. increased 3.7 years, from 34.7 to 38.4 years. This is higher than the national average of 37.6 years. Between 1991 and 2001 the number of seniors aged 80 and older increased dramatically from 87,065 to 134,175. This was a 54 percent increase and the highest level of growth in all the provinces.

One of the factors predicting the need for long-term care is the death of a spouse and the consequent loss of informal care. Senior women are much more likely to suffer the death of a spouse than men. Just over three-quarters (78 percent) of women 85 and over are widowed, compared to only 36 percent of men.

Living arrangements among seniors aged 85 and older also vary considerably by sex. Almost half (43 percent) of women 85 years old or older live alone. This is compared to 25 percent of men in the same age group. Similarly, almost one-third (29 percent) of women 85 years or older live in a health care institution. This is compared to 17 percent of men 85 or older.

### Entry to Long-Term Continuing Care
Admittance to RCFs is obtained through a single entry point system. Potential residents or someone on their behalf must apply by contacting the Home and Community Care Office of the local health authority. Depending on the level of urgency, a case manager will be appointed and an at-home assessment made. A care plan is designed and appropriate services provided, which may not necessarily involve residency at an RCF but could involve home support, home care nursing, palliative care, community rehabilitation, adult day centre, assisted living, residential care or hospice.

### Who Uses RCFs?
Residential care facilities target seniors with complex health problems, in particular Alzheimer's disease or other types of dementia. RCFs also target seniors who are physically dependent with medical needs caused by advanced age. RCFs are not exclusive to seniors, however, and may include younger adults with disabilities such as Parkinson's disease.

## The Yukon Territory
Long-term continuing care in the Yukon is delivered by Yukon Health and Social Services' Continuing Care Branch (CCB), which also delivers home care. The CCB describes the philosophy of care guiding residential care programs as follows:

> We are a community that respects and promotes dignity, individual freedom, choice and lifestyle, and meaningful quality living. We continually strive to create a feeling of home and belonging for all who live here by being responsive to the uniqueness of each resident. (YHSS 2007)

There are only three residential care facilities in the Yukon. Two (Copper Ridge Place and Macaulay Lodge) are located in Whitehorse and the third

(McDonald Lodge) services Dawson City. Below are brief descriptions of these facilities.

*Copper Ridge Place* is a 96-bed facility providing complex chronic care and extended care for individuals who require significant assistance with activities of daily living, monitoring and/or professional care on a 24-hour basis. Copper Ridge Place serves people of all ages, though it offers a special care program, providing individualized care for residents with dementia.

*Macaulay Lodge* is a 44-bed, intermediate care facility offering residential and respite care for both seniors and adults. The care levels provided at Macaulay Lodge are less intense than at Copper Ridge Place. The lodge targets individuals who require moderate assistance with the activities of daily living, monitoring and/or professional care on an intermittent basis throughout the day.

*McDonald Lodge*, located in Dawson City, is an 11-bed facility providing residential care to people who require light to moderate personal care, such as help with the activities of daily living, monitoring and/or professional care on an intermittent basis throughout the day. McDonald Lodge also offers home care nursing and home support services to people who live at home.

# 3

# Less Money, More People

## Implications of Policy Changes in Long-Term Care

Evelyn Shapiro and Morgan Seeley

In Canada, policy decision-making in regards to long-term residential care falls within provincial and territorial jurisdictions. The implementation of a number of recent policy changes by the provinces of British Columbia, Alberta and Manitoba should, therefore, be raising concerns about the impact of these long-term care reforms on the elderly, especially elderly women, who make up the majority of residential care users. The main goal of these policy changes is to spend less money on long-term residential care even as the number of elderly persons increases. By implementing a number of strategies, including reducing the number of long-term care beds in traditional care facilities, restricting access to 24-hour care and encouraging the development of "assisted-living" premises, these provinces are effectively downloading the costs of long-term residential care directly onto long-term care users.

This chapter explores some of the current policy changes to long-term residential care in British Columbia, Alberta and Manitoba. We argue that these changes will negatively impact the health and well-being of the elderly women living in or who need to live in these facilities, particularly those who cannot afford the cost of care and/or those who are vulnerable to losing access to services provided within long-term care residences. Similar changes are already occurring or are likely being planned elsewhere in Canada. It is therefore essential that this topic be placed at the top of research and political action agendas.

The provincial governments justify long-term care policy transformations in a number of ways. Concerns about the cost of a growing population of seniors to the health care system, what Gee and Gutman (2000) refer to as "apocalyptic demography," generate these funding and policy changes. This is despite the availability of health-policy research that challenges the notion of an aging population being primarily responsible for increased health care expenditures (Gee and Gutman 2000). Provincial governments also believe that the current and future cohorts of those aged 75 years or more will be wealthier than those who have gone before them. A report from the Premier's

Council on Aging and Seniors' Issues in British Columbia notes that "as a total population, older people in B.C. are better off financially than ever before, with higher incomes and considerable wealth in this group" (2006: 43).

Governments may see an opportunity to have users pay a greater share of the cost of their own care. What governments may not be considering is the economic inequality among seniors. For instance, in 2000, 75 percent of unattached women over 75 years of age — those who comprise the majority of long-term residential care users in B.C. — had annual incomes of less than $25,000 (Cohen, Murphy et al. 2005). While some seniors have greater incomes than previous generations, those who are most likely to require public long-term residential care are least likely to have the means to pay for it.

Policy changes to long-term care are also justified by reasoning that the younger elderly are healthier than previous generations and are also living longer, and may require help over a longer period of time as they become very old. Governments are therefore framing changes to long-term care policies as providing seniors with what they really want and need — namely, "more choices" and the opportunity of "aging in place."

Advocates of the expansion of for-profit long-term care facilities argue that for-profit facilities allow seniors and their families to evaluate various services and to choose the one that best suits their needs and interests. They also hold that market competition will ensure the provision of fiscally efficient, good-quality care (Pitters 2002). The concept of "aging in place" appeals to notions of deinstitutionalization. It promotes replacing residential care beds with assisted living and supportive housing and increasing access to home care in order to allow seniors to stay longer in their homes and communities. Yet the implications of long-term care policy changes in B.C., Alberta and Manitoba are troubling, particularly when the differential impact of these changes on particular groups of seniors, namely women and the most frail elderly, are considered.

In B.C., changes to long-term care are in full swing. The November 2006 Report of the Premier's Council on Aging and Seniors' Issues, which resulted from meetings with seniors across the province, noted that the numbers of nursing home beds have been and will be further reduced. These reductions reinforce more than a decade-long trend of mass closures to publicly funded long-term care residences and care beds across the province (Cohen et al. 2005). Long-term residential care beds are being replaced by a combination of some new nursing home beds, the closing down of other beds, the intro- duction of alternate assisted-living residential arrangements for those with less than 24-hour care needs, and increased home care resources. The report also notes that "this transition" does not appear to be going "smoothly." In fact, it says "there is great concern and scepticism" over whether the kind of residential care that elders need or can afford will be there when people need it (Premier's Council on Aging and Seniors' Issues 2006: 61).

It is also clear that women in particular will be affected. Since women on average live longer and are often sicker than men, there should be concern that long-term residential care services will not be there when they need them. Because women on average earn lower wages in the paid labour force, are over-represented in part-time and precarious work and are more likely to work at jobs with poor pensions and other benefits, women are less likely to have the economic resources needed to pay for care. Similarly, women's pensions are vulnerable to the time they lose in the paid labour force due to caregiving responsibilities, and many see their pensions reduced or cut if they outlive their partners or their partners divorce them (Premier's Council on Aging and Seniors' Issues 2006).

The Premier's Council also worries that, where the province needs to carefully match needs to services delivery, vulnerable elders are falling between the cracks. In addition to the overall reduction of existing residential care beds in B.C., plans for the development of new facilities and beds have largely been replaced by assisted living developments (Cohen et al. 2005).

Assisted living accommodations — where seniors who have daily care requirements live in their own apartments and receive care through the facility or through home care — might be appropriate for some seniors. Such services may permit seniors with low daily care needs to live in a setting more similar to a home than an institution, and maintain a greater sense of control and independence if they are able to make choices about the services they require and how their direct care will be provided. However, the shift from institutions to assisted living may turn out to be a loss of services previously provided by nursing homes. Alternate services may not provide what may be referred to as life-enriching activities, well-trained resources and quality care. The shift to assisted living may be particularly problematic for elderly women who do not have the financial resources to pay for appropriate, quality services when their needs are not thoroughly covered through assisted living arrangements. As Cohen and her colleagues argue, "Although the discussion [about assisted living] is framed in terms of the benefits of 'de-institutionalizing' care, the reality is somewhat different. The shift to an assisted living model may be more about limiting government's responsibility than about providing 'a homelike atmosphere'" (2005: 22).

In Alberta, a June 6, 2007, headline in the *Edmonton Journal* was "Changes in long-term care 'scary' for seniors." It decried that key medical and personal services were being "de-insured and privatized" as the province moves from nursing homes to "aging in place" care. Similar to the situation in B.C., a health policy focus of the Alberta provincial government is the expansion of long-term care services outside of residential facilities. The article also noted that the services previously provided by nursing homes were being "unbundled" by separating the costs of health from housing and support services, and limiting the available number of nursing home beds. The principles of the Alberta government's 2006 report outlining a ten-year plan for the future of continuing care in Alberta support this concern. The document prioritized unbundling services "so they can be delivered in a variety of sites" and implementing supports that will ensure "that Albertans can remain in their homes (their own house, apartment or supportive housing unit) for as long as possible based on "assessed needs" (Alberta Health and Wellness 2006: 4–5).

These "aging in place" strategies are not meant to work in conjunction with the development of much-needed long-term residential care facilities. They are designed to replace the demand for long-term beds. These strategies are made up largely of private, for-profit operations catering to clients who can absorb the cost of their own living arrangements and support care needs (Somerville 2007). For those who can't afford these costs, there is something called the Choice Program, which transports people to a day program in nursing homes in order to receive physician, nursing, therapy and medication management previously provided to residents in long-term care facilities. Some residential long-term care facilities are being converted to assisted-living centres, where vital personal care services such as feeding, hygiene and the administration of medications become a de-listed service under Medicare. In privatizing these medically necessary services, for-profit operators recover both operating and capital costs from the elderly end user.

A flood of letters to the editor of the *Edmonton Journal* followed the aforementioned exposé. Two headlines in particular struck us as interesting. One was "Aged care a growth industry for investors" and was subtitled "Government funding subsidizes profits from pensions of seniors." The second letter claimed that unbundling services for single long-term care residents with incomes over $23,000 would mean that they would be paying up to 75 percent of their before-tax income earnings for accommodation fees. This means a senior couple with a combined income of $36,000 would be spending 98 percent of their income for accommodation for both of them. By separating the costs of accommodation and health services within long-term care facilities, the cost of long-term care is effectively downloaded to the resident and/or her family. Furthermore, it provides for-profit investors with funds for which they are not accountable. This is particularly problematic given a preponderance of evidence suggesting that the expansion of for-profit long-term care facilities and related services does not ensure cost-effectiveness or good quality of care. The headline for another letter summed it up: "'Scary' is a mild term to describe the path this government is taking."

In Manitoba, a province with which we are more familiar, the Winnipeg Health Authority has just begun implementing its plan to close a substantial number of nursing home beds. Only a quarter of these units will be replaced with new, similar-type beds. To support this change, the Regional Health Authority has promised to provide more day spaces in the nursing home sector and more intensive resources for the home care program. The Authority has also approved and started the expansion of a model it refers to as Supportive Services for Group Living. These services are designed to provide enhanced support services to persons who already live in a community congregate setting, who do not require 24-hour support and supervision, but who are assessed as needing help with the instrumental activities of daily living. This model has been operating in a number of congregate settings for several years and has helped some persons return to or remain in the community for a longer period of time. Since most of these units accommodate persons living in government-sponsored, rent-to-income housing or non-profit housing sponsored by service clubs, ethnic or religious groups, the majority of units cater to elderly with limited incomes.

To deal with the closure of residential care beds, the Authority is also encouraging the development of a second service model, called supportive housing. Supportive housing initiatives target those elderly who require 24-hour support to live in the community. The sponsors, half of which are scheduled to be for-profit companies and the other half non-profit organizations, provide a housing and service package paid for by the tenants, while the Regional Health Authority funds and provides the nursing care component via home care. The housing and service package charges are substantial and, therefore, cater to seniors with incomes to match. However, for-profit owners are supposed to allocate ten units in each setting for lower-income elders, whose rent and service package will be subsidized by the Regional Health Authority.

Across the provinces of Manitoba, Alberta and B.C., provincial policy-makers are attempting to address the undersupply and increasing costs of residential long-term care facilities by substituting assisted-living and supportive housing services and promising to expand home care. We suspect that these types of plans and even their implementation are taking place quietly and without too much fanfare elsewhere across Canada, so their implications deserve attention. To add insult to what may turn out to be "injury," these changes are being sold to us (and who knows how many of us are buying into it) under the guise of giving us "more choices" or glorified visions of "aging in place." However, the substitution method does not rectify the undersupply of public long-term care facilities for a growing population of seniors. An overall lack of publicly funded residential, assisted and supportive housing units and services greatly impacts senior women, who comprise the majority of long-term care service-users. An undersupply of units and services mean that many senior women will have to turn to private, for-profit options to meet their care needs. This is particularly problematic for low- to middle-income seniors who do not quite qualify or who are waiting for access to residential long-term care services, but who are unable to afford private services or pay for a housing and service package that will ensure 24-hour support. While current policy changes to long-term care are supported by the notion of rising costs of care for the elderly population, Fuller, Fuller and Cohen suggest that "more and more low-income seniors will be left on their own to cope as best they can until a health crisis takes them to emergency and/or acute care" (2003: 18). Simply, an undersupply of facility-based long-term care beds means a sicker elderly population, which will result in an escalation of the costs to our health care system.

While assisted living and supportive housing may be an appropriate and positive option for seniors with low care needs and high incomes, it is not an appropriate replacement for residential care. There are significant problems related to the appropriateness, affordability and quality of care provided through assisted-living and supportive housing models. These substitutions tend to be made without consideration of the varying care needs of those more frail senior women, who might have access to residential care if such spaces were available.

Long-term care "options" are not good options for women when the quality of services provided are compromised. Unlike nursing homes, which are licensed and approved by provincial/territorial departments of health, currently, there is no apparent requirement for the government to ensure the quality of care provided in the assisted-living accommodations. There is no apparent requirement for the owners of assisted-living premises to provide staff training and supervision for the workers who are supposed to provide the support services for which residents pay the owners. The impact on residents is poor-quality care or the provision of care that does not meet their individual needs. Furthermore, women, as the overwhelming providers of paid care in these facilities, feel the impact when a lack of training and supervision means they are unable to provide the kind of care they know their clients need.

There is also no commitment on behalf of the provinces to ensure that these alternate living arrangements provide the life-enriching activities mandated for nursing home residents. The elderly may be pauperized by the charges levied for additional services or for the provision of day care. They may receive poorer services, or those who cannot afford the full service charges will not receive the services they really need. We are also concerned about the physical environment of alternate living arrangements. For those seniors with mobility impairments and chronic illnesses, more "community-based" supports and services may actually limit their engagement in everyday activities.

The privatization of residential long-term care options and the unbundling of long-term care supports and services from direct medical care (which occurs when nursing home units are replaced by outside options) are also problematic. The unbundling of services means that these services are no longer publicly insured. Not only does this mean that residents pay for services, but that these services will become privatized. Similarly, most of the new living arrangements in B.C. and Alberta and half of those in Manitoba will be owned by for-profit companies. A great deal of research in Canada has demonstrated that the privatization of health care services has a negative impact on women, who make up the majority of service users and providers. This body of literature suggests that private, for-profit services often provide poorer quality of care and that services become more costly. In this regard, we admit that we are not as concerned about those elders who have incomes well above the average, because many of them or their families are resourceful enough to move if they think the premises or the services they pay for do not meet their needs. But this is not the case with the majority of seniors, who have limited or low incomes. Additionally, private, for-profit services are less likely to employ unionized labour and are more likely to encourage higher profits by lowering workers' wages and failing to offer benefits and job security (National Coordinating Group on Health Care Reform and Women 2000).

Whereas nursing homes used to accommodate persons with similar needs for care, the new premises may produce ghettos in which each assisted-living or supportive housing arrangement houses persons with similar financial resources. This is clear in the case of Manitoba, where the development of supportive housing for low-income seniors and support services for group living for high-income seniors may be reinforcing health inequities among the elderly. The separation of seniors on the basis of income and care needs may end up affecting not only the quality of care that poorer elders receive but their quality of life. Furthermore, it is indeed possible that the very elderly, who have the most limited incomes and are, therefore, the least likely to be able to pay the additional costs associated with services, will receive poorer housing and/or poorer service delivery. In fact, we may get to the point where we witness a return to the old "rooming houses," which accommodated frail elders who were not quite poor enough to meet the provincial income criteria for help — something we thought we had eliminated a long time ago.

Although the provinces have indicated that they will increase the amount of home care resources to fill the gap resulting from the reduction in residential care units (nursing home beds), there is no formal commitment that this will happen to the extent needed. It is true that the provincial expenditures for home care have increased substantially over time, but the provinces must promise in advance to increase funding for home care for those elderly who choose to and can remain at home. But because long-term home care has always taken a back seat to post-hospital care, we have some doubts about the fulfillment of this promise. As we learned from the mass de-institutional-ization of people with disabilities across Canada, the closure of institutions was not met with the development or expansion of appropriate community resources.

We should also be aware that moving care back into the community and the home has a particular impact on women. Shifting from facility-based to home care means many of the costs of care are no longer covered by public insurance. In addition, limitations to the provision of paid home care mean that women, who provide about 80 percent of unpaid care, may experience increased demands on their time and resources. And women as paid provid-ers of home care are less likely to receive the quality of wages and benefits offered by public residential care facilities (for more information on women and home care, see National Coordinating Group of Health Care Reform and Women 2002).

For all these reasons it is important for us to find out what is going on in regards to long-term residential care, to assess the impact of these significant policy changes and to publish and publicize our findings. When we hear about the provinces and territories closing long-term care facilities and replacing them with assisted-living, supportive housing models and investments in home care, we need to be critical of claims to de-institutionalize seniors. Long-term care policy changes tend to be motivated by cost-cutting, not by attempts to increase the independence, health and well-being of seniors. This means that when we are promised "more choices" for "aging in place" we need to ask which seniors will have these choices and consider the ways in which the costs of long-term residential care are being downloaded onto women.

# 4

# A Contradictory Image of Need

## Long-Term Facilitative Care for First Nations

Nicole Eshkakogan and Nene Ernest Khalema

> There are deep and continuing disparities between Aboriginal and non-Aboriginal Canadians both in their overall health and in their ability to access health services. The reasons for this are complex and relate to a number of different factors, many of which have less to do with health and more to do with social conditions. (Romanow 2002: 211)

Why — when long-term care initiatives and policies promise care for all — are inequity of access, lack of integration of services and culturally incompetent services the norm for Aboriginal people[1] in Canada? This question forms the basis of this chapter, which aims to gain an understanding of the influence of policy on practice, to elucidate the social and historical discourses that exist about long-term care in First Nations communities and to draw out the commonalities and contradictions of long-term care policies as they relate to First Nations. It provides an overview of the context for the provision of long-term facilitative care for older First Nations in Canada and the contradictions between policy initiatives and service provision.[2] Drawing from the current literature, this chapter argues that long-term care as practised in Canada does not adequately address the specialized long-term health care needs of Aboriginal people. The planning and development of long-term care services for Canadians is underway, and it is imperative that Aboriginal people be provided the same access to resources and funding. They should not be overlooked because they have an atypical image and different long-term care service requirements than the majority of Canadians.

The chapter begins with a brief synopsis of Aboriginal demography and socioeconomic indicators, followed by a discussion of the long-term care needs of older Aboriginal people. Second, we draw attention to the areas of the Aboriginal population that have been significantly overlooked in terms of their long-term care requirements: Aboriginal children and youth with special needs, Aboriginal people with mental health challenges and Aboriginal people suffering from two or more chronic illnesses. Third, we contextualize the long-term care strategies in place for Aboriginal people and the associated perplexity in regards to funding and federal and provincial jurisdictional responsibilities. Finally, in response to the needs of Aboriginal people requiring long-term care, we recommend an approach that takes into consideration the context of health care provision and access issues; integration of services in terms of programming (i.e., stable, suitable and sufficient funding, the coordination of innovative and flexible long-term care service models and the development of a Aboriginal long-term care policy framework that will effectively negotiate jurisdictional responsibilities); and culturally competent long-term care services based upon Aboriginal values and practices.

## Information Synthesis and Analysis

Several electronic and library databases were accessed to locate existing research on long-term and continuing care issues affecting Aboriginal people. We found a paucity of research on this topic, and so we also relied on policies related to long-term and continuing care services for Aboriginal people, discussion papers, focus group meeting reports, conference minutes and non-academic papers to address this deficiency. While data about First Nations was limited, the most significant gap exists with respect to Métis, non-status First Nations, urban Aboriginal people and to a lesser extent, Inuit people. Therefore, most of the details and findings discussed in this chapter reflect those for registered First Nations.

## Aboriginal Demographic Trends and Epidemiological Indicators

The Canadian population is projected to age significantly as people are living longer and having fewer children. This is a significant demographic shift, and it is affecting the shape of the life cycle, the family and the ways in which we experience end-of-life. One significant change that is occurring is a shift in care needs; the incidence of acute illnesses in Canada is rapidly decreasing, while chronic, degenerative illnesses are on the rise. These factors all portend that formal care is going to be very important in the twenty-first century and that the incentives we create will strongly influence the way in which most people experience old age.

Compared to the general Canadian population the Aboriginal population is young, with 50 percent under the age of 25 years, and it is rapidly increasing in size, with the highest birth rate in Canada (RHS 2002–03). In 2000, Aboriginal women had a life expectancy of 76 years compared to 82 years for non-Aboriginals; and Aboriginal men's life expectancy was 69 years compared to 77 years for non-Aboriginals (Statistics Canada 2001). Thus, while the Aboriginal population is young, life expectancy is increasing and so is the population of older Aboriginal people.

In 2001, the on-reserve population of Aboriginal people aged 65 years and older was 28,200 (4 percent of the Aboriginal population). The latest projections indicate that the number of Aboriginal seniors is expected to grow more than two-fold by 2017, representing 6.5 percent of the total Aboriginal population (Statistics Canada 2006). In other words, the on-reserve Aboriginal senior population will increase to 59,500 by 2017. If we consider both on- and off-registered First Nations aged 55 years and older, the number more than triples to 138,435 by 2015 (Prince and Kelley 2006: 6).

Additional epidemiological data indicate that Aboriginal communities across Canada continue to face critical housing shortages, high rates of unemployment, lack of access to basic health services and low levels of education attainment. These broader determinants of health affect both life expectancy and quality of life for Aboriginal people. Compounded by broader determinants of health, epidemiological data also indicate that intentional and unintentional injuries are the leading causes of death of Aboriginal people, whereas circulatory system diseases account for the majority of Canadian mortality. Accordingly, Canada's Aboriginal people have the highest rates of morbidity, mortality and chronic disease. The principal causes of death for First Nations, Inuit and Métis are injuries, diseases of the circulatory system, neoplasms and diseases of the respiratory system (Smylie 2001: 3). The six most prevalent chronic conditions are arthritis or rheumatism, high blood pressure, asthma, stomach problems or intestinal ulcers, diabetes, and heart problems (Statistics Canada 2003: 4).

Many of the chronic conditions and illnesses that put First Nations people at risk of requiring continuing care begin to appear in the 45–64 year age group (Roscelli 2005: S56). In 1999, the leading causes of death among Aboriginals 45–64 years of age were ischemic heart disease (17 percent), lung cancer (6 percent), motor vehicle accidents (5 percent), diabetes (4 percent) and liver disease and cirrhosis (4 percent). The leading causes of death for Aboriginals 65 years and older were ischemic heart disease (20 percent), other forms of heart disease (9 percent), cerebrovascular disease (7 percent), lung cancer (7 percent) and pneumonia and influenza (6 percent). These trends reflect an epidemiological transition among Aboriginals that has been underway for more than 40 years and that consists of a shift from acute and infectious diseases to chronic and degenerative diseases associated with old age.

While the determinants of health are multifactoral, there is little doubt that Canada's Aboriginal communities have a great need for medical care (Kelly and Brown 2002; Prince and Kelley 2006). The demand for institutional and related continuing services for Aboriginals will grow rapidly over the next few decades due to the increases in the number of Aboriginals aging and the continuing disproportionate numbers of Aboriginal people of all ages requiring specialized care due to excess burdens of illness and mental health challenges.[3]

## Aboriginal Seniors

In the Aboriginal community, seniors are defined as those 55 years of age and older, because of their lower life expectancy and poor health (Health Canada 1998 cited in Dumont-Smith 2002: 6). The long-term and continuing care needs of Aboriginal seniors have long been ignored or minimized, due to the shorter life span of Aboriginal people (Prince and Kelley 2006: 6) or insufficient evidence (Bent 2004: 58). Almost no literature exists on older Aboriginals in Canada before 1985, unlike in the United States, where initial discussion and research dates back to the early 1970s (Buchignani and Armstrong-Esther 1999: 5). Several U.S. studies have focused on long-term, specialized and continuing care and Aboriginal people.[4] However, the service delivery systems, legal and political relations, demography, locales and living patterns of Aboriginal people in the U.S. are so different that American data is of limited relevance to Canadian contexts (Buchignani and Armstrong-Esther 1999: 7).

Regardless of racialization processes and geographic location, older people share complex needs because

- they are most commonly affected by multiple medical problems;
- the cumulative effect of these may be greater than any individual disease;
- they are at greater risk of adverse drug reactions and iatrogenic illness;
- minor problems may have a greater cumulative psychological impact; and
- problems of acute illness may be superimposed on physical or mental impairment, economic hardship and social isolation (WHO 2004: 14–15).

For older Aboriginal people, these complex needs are magnified by extreme poverty, rurality, poor housing, few household conveniences and limited transportation (Buchignani and Armstrong-Esther 1999: 21). For example, according to the First Nations Regional Longitudinal Health Survey (RHS) 2002–2003 report on First Nations seniors' health and well-being:

- over 40 percent of First Nations seniors have been affected by residential schools;
- First Nations seniors are nearly twice as likely as their Canadian counterparts to report one or more chronic health conditions (85.2 percent vs. 47.8 percent);

- arthritis affects 45.5 percent of First Nations seniors;
- nearly 80 percent of First Nations seniors rely on income from government sources;
- First Nations seniors have a median personal income of $12,991 and a median household income of $24,650; and
- almost half of First Nations seniors are in need of one or more home care services, and only one-third of those in need received care.

Literature on ethnicity and aging identifies cultural factors as a significant feature in understanding the availability and use of informal supports (Kreig et al. 2007: 12), and older Aboriginals have unique cultural orientations to consider. For instance, 79 percent of rural Navajo aged 60 and older expressed the need for help with wood hauling, 54 percent with wood chopping, and 45 percent with water hauling, activities essential to their survival in their particular cultural context but not common among the general elderly population (Jervis et al. 2002: 299). In their study on older Albertan Aboriginals, Buchignani and Armstrong-Esther (1999) found that very few of the seniors in their sample were financially prepared for independent living in old age or had the means to purchase private care of any sort. Yet, for the same sample, one in four seniors faced serious chronic physical or mental health difficulties requiring either institutionalization or high levels of informal care.

Magilvy and Congdon (2000) suggest that Aboriginal seniors are advantaged in the area of informal support due to community values and the importance placed on elders in Aboriginal culture. Many studies in the U.S. and a few in Canada have made the same assertion, advancing the notion that Aboriginal senior households therefore are rich potential sources of informal caregivers. However, Buchignani and Armstrong-Esther (1999) found that many Albertan Aboriginal seniors do not live in such households, residing instead either singly, with a spouse or with an adult child and grandchildren. Based on their study, they project a 50 percent increase in informal care responsibilities shouldered by Aboriginal community members over the next 20 years. Buchignani and Armstrong-Esther predict this increased load will fall disproportionately on women, which will have many implications for their other aspirations and obligations (1999: 15–25).

When we think of planning and developing long-term care services the need is mainly responsive to the trends in population aging. However, being "old" comes at different times to different people, and services should be developed around need rather than chronological age, diagnosis or other variables (Kite 2006: 459). This is especially true for Aboriginal people. Basic awareness of how history and culture have shaped the Aboriginal view of Western health care, and knowledge of the special problems and availability of resources for this vulnerable group are essential in providing Aboriginal people with safe and effective long-term care (Smyer and Stenvig 2007: 32).

And as proactive measures are needed to ensure that long-term care services are planned, developed and resourced to meet current and future population needs of older and aging non-Aboriginal Canadians, the same considerations must be made for Aboriginal people, who must not be disregarded due to their overall youthfulness.

## The Contradictory Image of Aboriginal Long-Term Care

Provincial reforms that occurred across the country throughout the 1990s have had a severe impact on First Nations health services and systems, adding to the uncertainty about what types of long-term care services should be provided for Aboriginal people living in various communities. This is compounded by the fact that the number of people requiring long-term care services is unknown.

Three areas of the Aboriginal population have been significantly overlooked in terms of their long-term care requirements. They are people who do not conform to the typical image of those in need of long-term care: Aboriginal children and youth with special health needs, Aboriginal people with mental health challenges and Aboriginal people suffering from two or more chronic illnesses.

Children's issues remain challenging to formal and informal caregivers. In some cases, children's health conditions deteriorate as they age, and eventually these children require higher levels of care (AFN 2005: 1). It is unclear how many children become wards of the child welfare system when they have to leave the community for specialized health treatment. Annual reports from provincial and territorial ministries of child and family services for the years 2000–2002 estimate that 76,000 children and youth are living in out-of-home care in Canada. An estimated 40 percent of these children are Aboriginal. Indeed, some provinces report that Aboriginal children comprise nearly 80 percent of children living in out-of-home care (Trocmé et al. 2004: 578).

The number of Aboriginal children placed in out-of-home care continues to rise. In fact, more Aboriginal children are placed in out-of-home care today than in residential schools at the height of the residential school movement (Trocmé et al. 2004: 579). The best sources of national data in Canada are the statistics kept by the Department of Indian and Northern Affairs (INAC), which funds child welfare services on reserves. INAC's year-end figures for children in care show a 71.5 percent increase in the number of on-reserve First Nations children in out-of-home care between 1995 and 2001 (Trocmé et al. 2004: 580). There is a great deal of variation across the regions in Canada with respect to administration and data collection. Although overrepresentation of Aboriginal children in out-of-home care is well documented, its explanation is unclear; thus the numbers of children who are in the child welfare system because of health ailments is not known. What is clear is that for children who remain with their families, most First Nations communities have no existing facilities and limited funding to respond to the specialized needs of diverse population groups, including children (AFN 2005: 2)

Brant (1994) identifies the following mental health issues in Native communities across Canada: widespread abuse of substances, including alcohol, solvent inhalation, street drugs and prescription medications; family violence, including spousal assault and sexual and physical abuse of children; and depression and hopelessness, often culminating in suicide. These issues are identified consistently across many Aboriginal communities in Canada (Smye and Mussell 2001: 7). Many of the mental health issues facing Aboriginal people today are rooted in historical and socioeconomic factors. Family violence, including physical and sexual abuse, is often the reason for referrals to mental health centres and hospitals and can be directly related to the historical legacy of Aboriginal people, such as the residential school system (Alberta Mental Health Board 2006: 24). For these reasons, the need for some specialized long-term care is due to the effects not just of mental illness, but of traumatic life experience.

Many Aboriginal people have suffered permanent brain injury as a result of trauma (accidents/assaults) or following long-term substance abuse (AFN 2005: 1). An unavoidable consequence that sometimes accompanies accidents, assaults and long-term substance abuse are disabilities, which also increase the demand for long-term care services. Given the fact that intentional and unintentional injuries and accidents are the leading cause of death for Aboriginal people, the revelation that Aboriginal people have higher rates of disability comes as no surprise. The disability rate among young adults is almost three times higher for Aboriginal people than for non-Aboriginal people. Sixty-six percent of Aboriginal adults with disabilities are affected by a mild disability, 22 percent by a moderate disability and 12 percent by a severe disability (AFN 2005: 1). The most commonly reported disabilities affect mobility, agility, and hearing and seeing (Smylie 2001: 9).

There are not enough resources to meet Aboriginal mental health concerns, in particular the needs of people affected by the residential school system (Smye and Mussell 2001: 3). There is a lack of timely, coordinated treatment and support for individuals with alcohol and substance use issues (in particular, across agencies and communities) as well as for people with serious mental illness who require immediate intensive care (Smye and Mussell 2001: 4). Alberta Health and Wellness and the University of Alberta Public Health Sciences (2004: 25) indicate that First Nations people seek help at higher rates than the general population for mental health problems, primarily through physicians, emergency rooms and hospital admissions rather than mental health outpatient clinics. Unfortunately, because many of these individuals are unable to access the necessary services to stabilize their mental health, they end up housed in correctional facilities. There is a desperate need to address this situation and seek alternative types of settings for these clients (AFN 2005: 2).

The prevalence of two or more chronic illnesses that limit independent living for Aboriginal people is increasing. For example, diabetes is expected to increase from 16 percent (1996) to 27 percent in 2016 (AFN 2005: 1). Aboriginal individuals with diabetes have high rates of complications and co-morbidities. Fifty-four percent of participants in the First Nations and Inuit Regional Health Survey (1999) who identified having diabetes also named having another chronic health condition (Smylie 2001: 6). Adults may also have two or more prevalent health conditions that further compromise their health (i.e., schizophrenia and a moderate to severe disability) (AFN 2005: 2). People with multiple chronic diseases or more than one prevalent health condition have poorer health outcomes and experience a greater need of health care resources. Furthermore, these individuals require more hospitalizations, longer hospital stays, more emergency visits and more time with family physicians and specialists. The costs and challenges of caring for this population are expected to rise due to the aging trend occurring within the Aboriginal population.

## Long-Term Care Strategies
## Implemented in First Nations Communities

Only 0.5 percent of First Nations communities have long-term care facilities (RHS 2002–03). This means that most Aboriginal people requiring care are placed in provincial/territorial facilities located outside of their communities — for some, a great distance away. Leaving the reservation for long-term care services makes Aboriginal people vulnerable to social isolation, depression and a decreased quality of life (Smyer and Stenvig 2007: 31). Two key programs were developed to address some of these issues: the First Nations and Inuit Home and Community Care (FNIHCC) program, set up by Health Canada, and the Assisted Living/Adult Care program, administered by Indian and Northern Affairs Canada (INAC). Both of these programs are limited to First Nations and Inuit communities, and do not offer services to Métis and non-status First Nations people, nor are they available to any status or treaty First Nations living in non-First Nations or Inuit communities.

The Assisted Living/Adult Care program consists of in-home care that provides homemaker services, foster care and institutional care limited to types I and II care of a non-medical nature to elderly or disabled First Nations living on reserves. Type I is institutional care for individuals requiring only limited supervision and assistance with daily living activities. Type II is extended care for individuals requiring some personal care on a 24-hour basis and those under medical or nursing supervision. However, the current policies, procedures and limitations of care within the INAC program exclude specialized care needs of other Aboriginal population groups (AFN 2005: 3). Of the 633 First Nations communities across Canada, only 30 communities have a personal care home (and these are limited to providing type I and type II care levels). INAC placed a moratorium on the construction of new care facilities in the late 1980s. This has since been lifted and replaced with very restrictive terms for approval of new facilities (AFN 2005: 3).

The FNIHCC program, launched by Health Canada in late 1999, is funded at $90 million a year and provides various health-related home care services, such as case management and nursing care (AFN 2005; NAHO 2002). The FNIHCC program spent approximately $36 million dollars on long-term institutional care in 2002–2003, which was provided through provincial or territorial institutions, but these funds are for low levels of care only. As of September 2003, the majority of eligible communities (96 percent) were being funded by the program, while 78 percent of eligible communities and 88 percent of the eligible population had access to full service delivery. In small and remote communities, however, even essential services are minimal due to lack of funds. In addition, there is some indication that the essential service elements are not always those that respond to the identified needs of the communities. The main ongoing gaps are perceived to be palliative care, rehabilitative care, respite care and mental health services (AFN 2005: 2–3). In addition, the FNIHCC program specifically excludes the construction of institutional long-term care facilities and the delivery of institutional long-term care services. This results in the sporadic provision of long-term care across First Nations and Inuit communities. The inherent problem of these service and funding gaps undermines the sustainability of the program and overextends staff. More importantly, First Nations and Inuit individuals requiring specialized long-term care services continue to be displaced from their communities to urban centres in order to receive the care they require.

Health Canada has maintained a strict policy of delivering health services only to registered status First Nations on reserves and has asserted that these services are a matter of policy, not a treaty right (MacKinnon 2005: S14). The federal government has taken the position that long-term care services for off-reserve First Nations, Métis and non-status First Nations should be covered by the provinces under the Canada Health Transfer (CHT). However, the provinces in most cases do not provide these types of services, citing federal constitutional responsibility (Roscelli 2005; AFN 2005). The discussions between federal and provincial governments to clarify jurisdictional issues over fiduciary responsibility for Aboriginal health care are ongoing — but without the involvement of Aboriginal people (Roscelli 2005: S57). It is through this jurisdictional interplay that the federal and provincial governments continually seek to find ways to make the other government pay the costs of services. Compounding jurisdictional and funding issues is the lack of current data that would highlight the costs of long-term care and end-of-life care needs for the majority of Aboriginal people and their communities. The First Nations Action Plan on Continuing Care (AFN 2005) puts the cost for continuing care expenditures not covered by federal jurisdiction at approximately $264 million annually.[5]

There is general agreement that the FNIHCC program and the Assisted Living/Adult Care program have responded reasonably well to the identified home care needs of Aboriginal people (AFN 2005: 8). However funding is spread too thinly, and the needs and appropriate long-term care service delivery systems are not well understood. What we do know is that in most Aboriginal communities there is next to nothing in the way of specialized long-term care that is specifically funded or mandated. Moreover, jurisdictional issues have become increasingly complex (NAHO 2002: 9) and can be a significant barrier for adequate and sustainable funding. Various funding issues need to be addressed to meet the increased demand and higher level care needs of those we have included in the contradictory image of long-term care, taking into account community size, location and other factors such as language, culture and requirements of the individual, family and community.

## Reducing Barriers

In order to effectively reduce barriers to long-term care for Aboriginal people, three issues need to be understood and addressed. These are lack of access to services due to jurisdictions, lack of integration of services and lack of cultural competency in provision.

Aboriginal people have unequal access to long-term care services because of jurisdictional issues that originate from conflicting constitutional responsibilities. For example, provincially funded programs often exclude status (registered within the *Indian Act*) and treaty (registered as a member of a tribe) Aboriginal people, living on and off reserve, because of "available" federally funded services. Additionally, services available on reserve are only for treaty Aboriginal people. Status and treaty Aboriginal people living off reserve do not have access to these federally funded programs. Status First Nations people have federally funded health services such as non-insured health benefits for prescriptions and dental care. These structural barriers make it difficult for First Nations communities to access long-term care services.

Lack of integration of services is also a major barrier in First Nations communities (Romanow 2002). Aboriginal funding for health services is "scattered among federal, provincial and territorial governments and Aboriginal organizations," complicating service provision (Romanow 2002: 217).

Integration of services is a daunting task. It can be a nightmarish experience to try to coordinate and document what funding is available and for whom. Given the overlapping responsibilities and the complexity of the health issues involved, better results could be achieved by sharing responsibilities rather than aggressively guarding jurisdiction (Romanow 2002: 221).

The inability of service providers to utilize culturally sensitive and culturally competent delivery models is also a major barrier in First Nations communities. Long-term care service providers appear to be ineffective in integrating Aboriginal ways of knowing about healing, recovery and death and dying.

## Community-Based Facilitative Long-Term Care

Emerging systems of community-based long-term care have been advanced to provide essential supports and services necessary to address the barriers mentioned above. According to Bartels, Levine and Shea (1999) home-and community-based long-term care models offer innovative approaches to providing medical and social services to older persons, yet they generally do not include specialized services for long-term mental health care of persons with severe and persistent mental illness. Bartels, Levine and Shea suggest that several examples of community-based long-term care — such as community-based intensive case management, 24-hour crisis intervention, home-based mental health care, residential and family support services, caregiver training and the use of multidisciplinary teams — have proved useful, especially in diverse communities. The outcomes for these programs indicate that with adequate supports, the majority of older persons can be maintained in the community at a lower cost than in institutions and with equal or improved quality of life (Bernstein and Hensley 1993).

To address First Nations' needs, a community-based long-term care facility requires community engagement and partnerships, not just to provide support for long-term care patients but as a way to build capacity in the community. But to ensure that Bartels, Levine and Shea's (1999) ideas are successful, especially in First Nations communities, the political will to provide stable, suitable and sufficient funding is necessary. This leadership by funding sources such as governments requires funding be matched to Aboriginal population growth, aging and to the specialized long-term care health needs of the Aboriginal population both on and off-reserve.

For on-reserve Aboriginals this might involve expanding the current FNIHCC program and the Assisted Living/Adult Care program to provide services of a medical nature (e.g., long-term rehabilitative and nursing facilities) as well as integrating existing support services (e.g., adult day care, respite care, personal care and boarding homes). For *all* Aboriginal people, regardless of ethnicity or geographical location, funding should support the coordination of innovative and flexible long-term care service models based upon shared Aboriginal traditional values, and opportunities where culturally specific approaches can be developed and implemented should be encouraged. Long-term care services compatible or congruent with cultural values and traditions and that ensure the likelihood of community involvement in planning and development are much more likely to be accessed (Levin and Herbert 2004: 168), and thus have a greater chance of effective service delivery and sustainability.

The multiple jurisdictional interplays between Aboriginal communities and the federal and provincial governments foil the collection of comprehensive and reliable Aboriginal health-assessment data (Smylie and Anderson 2006: 4). The long-term care needs of Aboriginals vary greatly depending on individual cases and disease progression, and it is important that the research agenda be broadened to take these into account. It is necessary to have accurate and reliable data upon which to form opinions about long-term care service needs and gaps. There is also a continued need for research on cultural and Aboriginal spiritual beliefs and practices (Prince and Kelley 2006: 8), which are fundamental to the development of specialized long-term care services for Aboriginal people. Developing and understanding long-term care from a diversity of Aboriginal perspectives may require adaptations to the current work in order to be in harmony with Aboriginal realities.

Aboriginal health planners, policy-makers and the different levels of government need comprehensive and reliable health-assessment measures that reflect the needs, priorities and understandings of health in their local and regional jurisdictions (Smylie and Anderson 2006: 605) to plan and develop an Aboriginal long-term care policy framework that will effectively negotiate jurisdictional responsibilities. The development of long-term care policy is essential for Aboriginal people both on- and off-reserve to ensure continuity of services and funding regardless of who is in power in government, band administration or bureaucratic levels or who holds management positions within the service delivery environment. Funding support for initiatives in service development, delivery and access remain inactive without policy direction in long-term care.

If long-term care services are to provide choice, and be flexible and responsive to the needs of Aboriginals, there will need to be integration across the whole sector. This will require a range of partnerships. It will also require innovative thinking and action to assist in building communities with the capacity to respond to the needs of those with a long-term illness, their families and service providers. Creating this community capacity also requires recognition of its limits. Significant progress has been made over the last decade, and there are longstanding and newly emerging advances and strengths in the current system that provides long-term care services to Aboriginal people. Building on those strengths, an agenda for next steps towards long-term care policy that addresses all Aboriginal people needs to be created. All of these efforts will require financial resources. Lacking these, Aboriginal people and their communities will likely continue to find themselves going without much-needed long-term care services.

## Notes

1.   This chapter uses both Aboriginal and First Nations interchangeably. Aboriginal is used in Canada to include non-status and status Indians, Métis and Inuit (all legal terms) as defined by the *Constitution Act* 1982. Indian is defined by the federal *Indian Act* as a person who is registered as an Indian or is entitled to be registered as Indian. We use the term First Nation(s) to refer only to those Aboriginal people who are entitled to be registered as Indians, and to refer to the reserve that those people are from.

2.   Our work is framed by understandings derived from Indigenous ways of knowing and doing, which directs attention to the web of social, spiritual, political and economic relations surrounding individuals and social groups. We stress that this framework should not be interpreted in a crudely deterministic and essentialist fashion, which neglects the nuances of diversity and agency within First Nations communities in Canada. For more information about the approach we have adopted, see Browne and Smye (2002).

3.   It is well understood and documented that the current health status of Aboriginal people is deeply rooted in severe disparities of health determinants such as poverty, social exclusion and lack of education. Governmental policies of assimilation (The *Indian Act*, the residential school system and child welfare policies) have tragically weakened other important determinants such as social support networks, parenting skills, personal health practices, coping skills and traditional culture.

4.   Buchignani and Armstrong-Esther (1999) cite Versen 1981; Strong 1984; Weibel-Orlando 1989; Hennessy and John 1995; Robert John 1985, 1986, 1990, 1991; Randy John 1995; and Kramer 1991.

5.   Specifically, the AFN notes: "Although there is limited data on the continuing care needs of First Nations, a rough estimate on the cost for First Nations has been determined based on the cost of providing services to the average Canadian public, with adjustments for factors specific to most First Nations communities such as remote location, health status (i.e., high prevalence of chronic and infectious diseases) and diseconomies of scale. It is estimated that the total cost of home care and institutional care for First Nations communities and settlements would be in the range of $430 million annually. This amount would be reduced by the total estimated annual expenditures of the existing programs provided by Health Canada and INAC, which is $166 million, resulting in an estimated cost of $264 million. This estimate would be further reduced by the amount that the provincial government may contribute to the higher levels of care for First Nations but no specific information is available regarding provincial expenditures. As stated, provincial services to on-reserve residents are minimal" (AFN 2005: 6).

# 5

# A Dream Retirement Community

## Long-Term Care Options

Beverly Suek

I have often been accused of being an incurable optimist. I believe we can change the world and make a difference. Sometimes I'm right, and sometimes I'm a bit… disappointed.

In terms of long-term care for women, I have a dream — which I hope will one day become a reality.

There have been a number of steps along the way to envisaging this dream. In fact, a few years ago, I didn't give it a thought. Becoming a senior seemed very far away. I have seven children, and I had made it clear to them that I had every intention of making them take care of me in my advanced years.

But one realization, which gets stronger the older I get, is that I don't want to be under the care and control of my children and their partners. I want to be with friends my own age — people who actually remember Doris Day and Rock Hudson and know that the Big Bopper is not a jump toy.

Another realization hit me when my mother went into long-term care. She remarried at 80 and had six glorious years with her new partner, until she had a stroke. She needed care — physical care. The choices were a private facility where both she and her partner could live, for $6000 a month — or subsidized care, where she would be institutionally separated from the love of her life. They didn't have $6000 a month, so he lived in one place and she lived in another. We're told that we live in a world where we support families, but in fact we separate them in the way we set up long-term institutional care.

This was a huge change in her living arrangements, but to add to that, my mother was also "locked in" the building. Because many of the home's residents were living with dementia, none of the residents was permitted to leave unless accompanied by an adult — which it was assumed they weren't.

She had no choices in terms of when she got up, when she had lunch, what she had for lunch or when she went to bed. These simple decisions were no longer hers to make. They were made by strangers who did not take into account her individual preferences.

She was in a two-bedroom suite that she shared with a woman who had dementia and was unable to communicate, adding to my mother's sense of loneliness.

For me as a family member, visiting was not a loving and caring experience. I longed to be alone with my mother and to have a double bed where I could lie down with her, hug her and hear her tell her life stories, uninterrupted. I would have loved a little couch where we could sit together and watch something inane on TV and laugh together. But what we had was one hard-backed chair and little opportunity to touch or be close.

My mother died in this long-term care facility with eight of us crowded around her bed, while her roommate tried to sleep. It was not the end-of-life transition I would have hoped for her.

Her experience brought the long-term care issue home to me, in terms of what is available in the real world. I had not known before the reality of what exists today. Many of us have experienced a similar situation with loved ones, but it is an individualized event, burdened by sadness. So far, we have not rallied together to shout out loud that "this is not good enough!" Is this the respect and caring that seniors deserve in their final years?

I also wondered what it would be like for me, when I need long-term care. Will there be options? Will I have a say in where I live? Will I have control over my own living environment?

And what about my friends who are in lesbian relationships? Many non-profit long-term care facilities are run by church groups or charities. If heterosexual couples are having trouble staying together in long-term care, I wondered what the situation would be like for homosexual couples.

So about three years ago, a group of us got together to clarify our dreams and discuss how we could make a difference. We wanted to define a new set of principles and values congruent with women's lives and redesign retirement homes and long-term care facilities. (For us, retirement housing and long-term care are one and the same, as our concept includes complete continuity of care, rather than the current practice of having to move from one type of facility to another as seniors need more assistance with daily living.) Our ultimate goal was to get financing and actually build a retirement village for women — to construct a prototype that could be used elsewhere.

Our group was diverse — made up of Aboriginal women, immigrant women, women with family members with disabilities, lesbian women and heterosexual women. It was co-chaired by singer and songwriter Heather Bishop and me. We called ourselves the Committee for Retirement Alternatives for Women.

After several meetings, we defined our main objective: to develop affordable housing that is sensitive to an active and diverse female community. We agreed that the retirement housing would be built on principles of respect, diversity and community building. Here is our set of principles.

We believe

- that the housing should support a sense of community, with people helping people, sharing and caring;
- that the housing should be integrated into the community at large, not isolated;
- that the housing will be built with environmentally friendly features and will operate with minimal negative impact on the environment;
- that there is respect for the experience and knowledge of the residents and their knowledge should be passed on to others;
- that respect for differences will be a key principle, with a conflict resolution mechanism to resolve disputes;
- that diversity will be a principle and be inclusive of the needs of women from different cultural backgrounds, Aboriginal women, lesbian women and women with disabilities;
- that the governance model will allow for participation of the residents in the policies and operation of the housing complex;
- that individual residents will have control over their living environment;
- that there will be options for women to choose to participate in programs, to have privacy, to interact with others, to interact with the community, to travel, etc.;
- that there should be a continuity of care, from early retirement housing to comprehensive care, at the same location; and
- that the housing should be affordable for access for low-income women.

These principles include our aims for both retirement housing and long-term care — for both when we're able-bodied and when we have impediments of various kinds and need more care. We see ourselves as helping one another, creating a community where we care about and for one another to the best of our abilities, and where we don't ship some women off to another institution because they need greater care. Our dream has to include both.

## Affordable Housing

Let's face it; many women over sixty are poor. I have two sisters — both stayed home with their kids for twenty years and, as "unemployed" homemakers, couldn't pay into the Canada Pension Plan. One sold real estate and had no pension. Later, she got a part-time job with no pro-rated pension. The other went back to work when her children were older but only had a few pensionable years and ended up with such a small pension that it wouldn't cover the cost of a room at the YWCA. Both got divorced but didn't receive support payments for themselves. They are not the exceptions.

Many women have no pension. Those who counted on their husband's pension but are now widowed have discovered that they are only entitled to two-fifths of what their husband received.

If anyone thinks that private, for-profit retirement housing will meet the needs of women, they better rethink.

## Not Just Housing But Community

We're not just talking about housing; we're talking about building communities. One of the dilemmas for seniors is loneliness. Your children are grown up and busy with their own lives. They call and they email, but they have their own issues to deal with. Some of your friends and siblings are in long-term housing or have died. Many women chose to stay in their own home for as long as possible, to retain control of their lives, but find that they have limited social interaction. Getting out, particularly in winter, is difficult, and it becomes easier and easier to stay home. But the isolation leads to a life of loneliness.

Our dream is to design a housing alternative that allows for control over individual decisions but also offers the option to have company. We want a design that encourages both conversation and cooperation.

Heather Bishop built a small replica of the retirement village out of tin cans and cardboard to get a better picture of what our dream might look like. The village has two floors with an enclosed inner courtyard. There could be anywhere from 30 to 150 suites — some one-bedroom and some two-bedroom, to accommodate single people and couples. Each suite will also have a living room and a small kitchen area and an outdoor balcony, preferably screened in to stop those pesky mosquitoes.

There's an internal walkway on both the first and the second floors, where women can sit outside their rooms, have tea and chat to people who walk by or watch the art or tai chi classes. The centre will have a café serving excellent coffee as well as a common kitchen, where women who feel so inspired can cook for others when they want to.

There will be accommodation for families who come to visit and they will be made welcome.

A portion of the building will be dedicated to women who need intensive care, but they will still be part of the community.

Retirement housing is often built on the outskirts of cities and towns where there is no access to stores or movies or decent coffee house and restaurants. This is particularly inhospitable to seniors who have stopped driving. We see our retirement housing as being an integral part of a larger community. Our design has a front section that is like a community centre, with a pool that can be used by the community as well as by us, and rooms for residents to use their knowledge and experience to teach anything from knitting to economic theory.

We'd like the recognition that we have wisdom and talent to share with the community.

As well as wisdom, we have a capacity for caring for one another. Too often when a friend becomes disabled or is dying, our first thought is to send them off to the health professionals. But for us, the retirement village is as much about caring for one another as it is about housing. I'm not talking about doing heavy lifting or emptying bed pans, but developing a sense of community where we can offer a hand in a time of need.

Several years ago, our eldest son died of AIDS. When he became gravely ill, we could no longer provide all the care for him at home. A group of friends got together and took turns providing care at home, so we could spend time with him. It was a gift from them to help us, but it was also a gift to them from him, to let them into his life and share this final transition with them. We went on to form an organization to help people with AIDS stay at home and, if it were their choice, to die at home. This can be done. It's not for everyone and it too would be a choice. But for those who are willing and able, caring for our neighbours would be an essential part of our community.

## Control of Our Lives

When I talk to women, they say that the single most important aspect of seniors' housing is housing that provides as much control over their lives as they can manage.

We do not want just to be taken care of, we want to participate. We are Baby Boomers who were brought up on the patriarchal mindset of *Leave it to Beaver* and *Father Knows Best*. We moved on to reading Betty Friedan and Germaine Greer and taking to heart Erica Jong's *Fear of Flying*. We fought to change the society we were living in and to have more control over our own lives as women. We're not planning on giving up the control we've worked so hard for.

We want to live where we can decide to sleep in until 10 a.m. if we want. We want to decide to play chess with a friend or watch old Katherine Hepburn movies until 2 a.m. We want to have double fudge chocolate cake rather than jello for dessert. We want to have a big bed where we can snuggle with our loved ones.

And we actually want to run the place, not be subject to a board of directors made up of guys in suits. We understand that some of us may not be able to participate fully, but others, who may be physically incapacitated, will continue to be mentally competent.

## Making the Dream a Reality

The first challenge is to change the premise on which we create long-term care. I had a "eureka" moment at the Designing Long-Term Care with Women in Mind workshop when Marta Szebehely of Sweden (see Chapter 9), suggested that in Canada, we conceptualize long-term care on a health care model, not a housing model. While most retirement homes have some of the qualities of a home, when we switch to long-term care, we build hospitals, not homes. There's a nursing station, limited visiting hours, long corridors with institutional decor, often two to four beds in a room, like hospital wards. There is no privacy and the schedule is determined by a pre-set timetable, not by the wishes of the resident.

What if we changed that premise? What if we recognized that, although some seniors may be incapacitated, this is their home, and probably the last one they will know? What if we built them as homes for seniors, with health care directed at their needs as an added service to them? What would long-term housing look like then?

## Options

To paraphrase Heather Bishop, this may be another example of feminist women working to change the world, where we push open a new door, but never get to walk through ourselves. So as we work for change for the future, what are our options now?

### Build Our Dream Retirement Community

Being an incurable optimist, I will continue to work towards the dream of a perfect retirement village for women, however impossible it may seem.

As a committee, we have done a lot of research to find funding sources. We have applied for grants, but housing grants have their own impediments. For one provincial grant for non-profits, you have to purchase the land and complete an architectural drawing before you can even apply. It is designed for large non-profits with substantial resources, not for underfunded women's groups. One of the people assessing our grant application suggested that we ask women's organizations to provide start-up funding. But how many crisis shelters and women's groups have excess funding? We've been turned down three times for housing grants already, but we'll keep trying.

In researching this option, we tried to find similar concepts elsewhere. We were unable to find a women's retirement community anywhere in Canada. We did, however, locate one in Carefree, Florida. Heather Bishop was invited to sing there and I joined her as her "roadie."

Carefree is a gated, all-women community near Fort Meyers, Florida <www.carefreecommunity.com>. It was originally started by two women. It grew out of a group of women who travelled frequently in recreational vehicles (RVs) and would join up in warm places to park their RVs and be together with like-minded women. This evolved into the building of about 200 modular homes in Carefree, most with parking for an RV. It has a clubhouse with a variety of facilities and activities. Although it wasn't intended as a retirement community, many of the residents have now retired to Carefree. Most are over 50 and most are lesbian couples.

It was marvellous staying in a community of women — women driving around in their golf carts or walking their dogs along the streets. One of the women we met was suffering from early dementia, and it was interesting to see how she was treated. She was invited to the potlucks and would tell a story over and over again, or say something out of context, but everyone was caring and respectful, and she was fully part of the group.

The village seems to work well for them, but it appeared to be missing some of the key principles of our dream. Because of how it evolved, it was not set up for retirement and there is no long-term care plan. One woman had a stroke and was being moved out to a long-term facility, away from the village. The individual houses with no front porches did not lend themselves to casual interaction. There were, of course, events organized at the clubhouse and group potlucks, but not the ongoing community interaction that we envision.

There was controversy about when and how to allow men and male children on the site, with some wanting no males at all, others wanting them to have more access and others somewhere in the middle. Having sons and a grandson of my own, I would certainly be on the easy access side myself, but it is a question that will arise with women-only retirement villages.

However, the women who live at Carefree do have control over their community environment and their individual living space. It is a wonderful experiment that they have created and one that we can learn from.

## Build Small Retirement/Long-Term Care Housing in Communities

I live in an old neighbourhood in Winnipeg called Riverview. An older couple who used to live two doors down are in long-term care on the other side of the city, away from the friends and neighbours they've known all their lives. Their house has been vacant for over two years. They still hope to return to the community, however unlikely that may be.

We have an aging population in our neighbourhood who will face a similar choice. Why not learn from many rural towns, who build housing for seniors to keep them in their own communities? Let's build housing for seniors which is integrated into urban communities and incorporate art classes for kids, playgrounds, soccer fields and play activities for adults to interact with senior adults and bring back the concept of community.

While this is not an exclusively women's option, it is another way of conceptualizing retirement housing.

## Stay in Your Own Home as Long as Possible

For many women, staying in their own home is the preferred option, because there are currently no others that give us the independence and control we seek. When I talk to older women about this, they often say, "I'm fine in my house. I manage quite well." They don't want to talk about what will happen if they have a stroke or break a hip or become forgetful. No one wants to talk about that.

But we must talk about it.

Some provinces are increasing their home care services in anticipation of the baby boomers choosing this option, and that's good for those who make this choice. But the big downside is loneliness. You live alone. It takes effort to call a friend to go to a movie, to arrange transportation or to walk down an icy path to a taxi. Many women just stop doing it because it's too difficult. They find themselves isolated and lonely.

Some will make the effort and this option will work for them and should be supported with home care services. Others may choose to have more of a community around them, and this too should be an option.

## Live with Your Relatives

I know one woman and her daughter who are both pleased with their plan to live together. This option may work for people like them, with the additional support of home care to lighten the burden on family members.

For others, this is neither an option nor a preferred arrangement. I have wonderful children, and I think I could coerce one of them into taking care of me — guilt would probably work. But the question is, would I like it? Having been the person that they depended on for their younger years, I don't know that I'd ever be ready for a role reversal, where I would be the dependent one.

I've always thought that the hardest lesson for us — as feminists who have been so fiercely independent — is to learn to ask for help, to admit to some dependence. But if this is a lesson I have to learn, I think it would be easier to learn it from my friends than from my children.

Love them I do, but live with them? I don't think so.

And many women have no children or other relatives, so this not an option for them at all.

## Private Retirement Housing

If money is not a problem, a retirement home is an option. But for most women, pension income and assets are limited. I recently visited a private retirement home, and the one-bedroom suites started at $600,000. This is not within my budget nor within the budgets of most other women.

It was classy. Marble counter tops and state-of-the-art fixtures. The building had a common room with a pool table and a place to watch TV together. But the focus was more on recreation than building community and more on entertaining seniors than creating an environment of respect for their knowledge and experience. There was no provision for them to participate in the decision-making of the operation of the complex. And it was located in an area too far for any but the most energetic seniors to walk to restaurants or grocery stores.

If I did have $600,000 to spend, I think I would choose one of the following options instead.

## Create Your Own Retirement Community

Why not? I've talked to some women who are considering pooling their savings with four or five other women to buy a large house and convert it into individual suites. An additional suite could be for a staff person to help when help is needed.

Others are talking about buying a small apartment block and doing the same thing. Years ago, a group of eight women, including me, bought a 12-suite apartment block in Wolseley, Winnipeg's granola belt. We set it up as a cooperative, with the intention of making it our future retirement housing. None of us had bought an apartment block before but found it quite easy to do. We made the two basement suites into a common area and the people living in the block could have privacy, or could leave their doors open and have company. Two of our group moved in, but later left, and the existing co-op members now own the building (long story made short). Simply put, we made some errors in the organizational structure, but it was a good idea then, as it is now.

Heather Bishop started a land cooperative years ago, with several women getting together to buy land in the country and build their own homes on the land. They too had a solid agreement so that all understood the terms and how to get in and how to get out of the cooperative. Heather still lives there happily with her partner.

There are a number of organizational structures that could work for women considering creating their own retirement options. It could be a co-op, it could be a corporation with partners or shareholders, or it could be a sole proprietorship if one person had the money and the others were renters. There are two important items to consider. One is that you need an excellent agreement between the parties in advance about the values and principles, who is a member, how members can get their investment out and how to resolve conflict. The other is a monthly payment that includes enough for maintenance and upkeep so that you're not stuck short when the roof leaks.

Until we actually get changes in the existing retirement and long-term care options, or a women's retirement community, we may have to depend on our own creativity and initiatives to create our own.

## What We Want

First, here's what we don't want for our future. We don't want to make Styrofoam snowmen to keep us busy. We don't want to be warehoused in quad rooms down long hallways where there is no interaction with other residents. We don't want to be loaded with tranquillizers and sleeping pills to keep us quiet.

I don't want the limited choices that my mother had. I wish she had had more choices and I wish that I had done more to make her final years in long-term care better. I wish that I had crawled into her single bed and hugged her, even if it was against the rules. I wish that I had visited more or stayed longer, even though I found the environment inhospitable. I wish that I hadn't placidly obeyed the rules. There was one time I did not. My mother was dying and the staff wanted to send us home because visiting hours were over. I refused to leave and slept several nights in that hard-back chair. I am glad of that one recalcitrant act, because my best memory is of her waking up, looking over, seeing me, smiling and squeezing my hand. It was the last time I saw her lucid and it means the world to me.

I can't make it different for her. But I can do whatever I can to make it different for me, for my wonderful sisters, for the friends I love dearly and for future generations.

What we want for ourselves and others is respect in our senior years. We want control over our living environment. We want companionship of people our own age, as well as interaction with all generations. We want to remain part of the community.

We don't want to be quiet! We want to shout loudly, be cantankerous when we need to be and love when we can. We want to continue, as we always have as women, to live life fully and bravely.

# 6

# A Failure of Vision and Political Will

## The Reality of Long-Term Care in Ontario

Sheila Neysmith

Albert Banerjee's overview of long-term care in Canada (chapter 2 in this volume) ably highlights some of the dynamics in the long-term care policy field in Canada. Of the five regions that he presents, Ontario merits the harshest description: "In sum, according to the PriceWaterhouseCoopers survey, Ontario long-term care residents are among the oldest, have one of the highest rates of mental impairment and are the most depressed." "Challenging Questions," by Pat Armstrong, with Albert Banerjee (chapter 1 in this volume) clearly indicates that the people behind the statistics are predominantly women. Furthermore, Pat argues that one of the underlying dynamics at work in Canada is that using the long-term care system is seen as a failure: a failure of family, of individuals, of women and of care.

In this chapter, I argue that the real failure is not at the level of individuals receiving or providing care — rather it is a failure of policy vision and political will. Real vision would mean placing long-term care facilities within a broader policy of community-based services where women people the policy stage. Assessing policy options would mean using a gender lens while recognizing that policies have differential impacts on women, who, at any particular historical moment, might be situated as care receivers, paid providers or family members. Although my remarks are rooted in the Ontario reality, designing long-term facility care with women in mind is a Canada-wide challenge.

Three main themes underlie my discussion of the situation of long-term care in Ontario. The first is that long-term care policy continues to be a response to crises in acute care. One such response, popularly referred to as early discharge, effectively reduces costs to hospital budgets. However, costs do not disappear; rather public costs are turned into private costs as families, usually female kin, pick up the necessary but unpaid care work. For instance, the Canadian Home Care Association identified acute, not supportive or chronic, home care as its priority area for 2004–2005. Provincial equivalents of Ontario's Community Care Access Centres (CCACs) and Quebec's Health and Social Service Centres (CSSSs) had little choice but to prioritize their limited budgets towards patients discharged from hospitals who still needed intensive services at home. The Ontario government's policy statement *Commitment to Care* (Ontario 2004) and its subsequent funding of long-term care beds were in part motivated by the need to relieve pressure on acute care beds occupied by chronic care patients, referred to as "bed blockers."

Second, the proliferation of retirement homes masks a crisis in supportive housing, which has been ignored by all levels of government for the last decade and a half. The shortage of supportive housing is more critical for women because we live longer and typically earn less so are less likely to be able to afford upper-end retirement homes. Third, policy inaction can all too easily be justified by invoking myths that in culturally diverse urban centres, families are able to care for relatives with even high levels of need because placing a family member in long-term care is considered a disgrace. Missed in this stereotype is the fact that in most communities it is women who do the actual caring work as wives, daughters, daughters-in-law or as volunteers in various faith-based or cultural communities.

## Seniors' Residential Options in Ontario

In Ontario, three main types of residential settings provide both accommodation and care for seniors: supportive housing, retirement homes and long-term care homes. Table 6.1 illustrates the options available to seniors.

### Retirement Homes

There are more than 41,000 seniors living in Ontario's 700 retirement homes. It is important to underline that, unlike nursing homes, these residences are not regulated. Living in one is essentially like living in an apartment or hotel. Retirement home residents pay for their own care and accommodations. Retirement homes may be an option for people who have the resources to rent within the luxury market, but even there it is a situation of "buyer beware." Because they are in the private market, information is spotty. In 2007, Canada Mortgage and Housing Corporation did a survey of the Ontario market but the information was limited to the size of complexes, types of suites available, their geographical distribution and monthly costs (CMHC 2007). There was no information on, for example, the numbers of men and women residents. However, since many women have limited incomes in old age, it is safe to assume that they were in the lower end of the market.

A Retirement Home Consultation carried out between January and March 2007 recommended that the Ontario government

- establish mandatory province-wide standards;
- establish a new agency, independent from government, to enforce these standards;

**Table 6-1: Seniors' Care: Comparing Residential Care Options**

| Types of Residential Accommodation | Retirement Homes | Supportive Housing | Long-Term Care Homes |
|---|---|---|---|
| Also Called | Retirement residence, Care home, Assisted living, Rest home | Non-profit housing, Social housing, Seniors' housing | Homes, Nursing homes, Homes for the aged |
| Levels of Care | Meals, light housekeeping, low levels of personal care and availability of staff on a 24-hour basis | Daily personal care, 24-hour availability of a trained personal support worker, meal preparation and/or homemaking | For those who need higher levels of daily personal care, availability of 24-hour nursing care or supervision, and a secure environment |
| Ownership and Management | Private for-profit corporations and in a few cases, non-profit corporations. | Building management varies. Services managed by non-profit corporations | Municipal governments, non-profit corporations or private for-profit corporations |
| Cost Ranges (Per person) | Costs for accommodation and care can range from $1500 to $5000 per month for a private room | Costs range from $600 to $1200 per month. Rent subsidies are sometimes available. Support service costs are covered by MOHLTC | $1543.95 per month for "standard or basic," $1787.29 for semi-private, $2091.45 for private |
| Government Funding | None | Government can subsidize rent to the level of 30% of gross household income. MOHLTC funds support services | Government subsidizes the "basic or standard" rate for those who qualify. MOHLTC funds the care provided in homes |
| Governing Legislation | *Tenant Protection Act*. Some municipalities may also have "care home" bylaws. | Building tenancy: *Tenant Protection Act*; Service provision: *Long-Term Care Act* | Bill 140, *An Act Respecting Long-Term Care Homes* (June 2007) |

*Source: Adapted from the Ministry of Health and Long-Term Care (MOHLTC) website*

- build on the existing voluntary standards of the Ontario Retirement Communities Association (ORCA), refined over the past 13 years; and
- provide education and training for all retirement home staff so they can understand and meet the new service standards.

In response to these suggestions, the government is conducting a survey to determine the level of care and services being purchased by residents of Ontario's retirement homes. It is also consulting stakeholders on what should be included in a standard, plain-language contract between retirement homes and residents. The new contract will detail what care and services are being purchased and will inform consumers and their families about alternative, publicly funded services to help ensure they make informed choices about their care and accommodation options. At present the Ministry of Health and Long-Term Care (MOHLTC) website offers only a guide and tips for touring a residential setting. Although such initiatives are welcomed, the gender-neutral language of "stakeholder" suggests that a gender-based analysis will not be forthcoming.

While the debate about the quality of so-called retirement homes and seniors' villages flourishes, the dearth of supportive housing is ignored. To put it bluntly, focusing on improving retirement homes distracts from undertaking much-needed action around supportive housing.

## Supportive Housing

Supportive housing is "housing plus support." It is designed for people who need minimal to moderate care — such as homemaking or personal care and support — to live independently. Accommodations usually consist of rental units within an apartment building. In a few cases, the accommodation is a small group residence.

People typically need support when they are

- chronically homeless and hard-to-house;
- frail elderly;
- physically disabled;
- developmentally disabled;
- seriously mentally ill;
- victims of violence;
- living with HIV/AIDS;
- youth; or
- have substance abuse problems.

As Table 6.1 shows, supportive housing buildings are owned and operated by municipal governments or non-profit groups, including faith groups, seniors' organizations, service clubs and cultural groups. Accommodations, on-site services, costs and the availability of government subsidies vary with each building. The care arrangements between a tenant and a service provider are usually defined through a contract between the two parties. Although technically the for-profit sector could be a provider, the retirement home market has far more profit potential.

Bringing a gender lens to bear on retirement homes and supportive housing reveals several troublesome dynamics that affect women. First, upper-end retirement home advertisements present a lifestyle image that assumes a retired couple. Demographically that is a short phase in most older women's lives. Divorce, death and deteriorating health — the realities that many women face — are not part of this image. Although some women will have command of sufficient financial resources throughout their lives, these are the minority and not the focus of supportive housing policy. Second, a gender lens analysis would ask, who are the people living in the lower-end retirement homes? Who is living alone in the community? What factors affect older women's decisions to enter a retirement home? Who are the women in such settings? Third, what kinds of supports do these women need? Who will provide this? What are the implications for service providers — most of whom will be women?

Supportive housing has been neglected across the board in Ontario since the election of the Mike Harris Conservative government in the mid-1990s. There are now some attempts to resuscitate it, but it will take a lot of hard work. For one thing, the infrastructure has greatly deteriorated. For instance, a 2007 report released by the Ontario Non-Profit Housing Association (ON-PHA 2007) stated that a third of executive directors in the non-profit housing sector would retire over the next five years with nobody in the pipeline to replace them.

## Long-Term Care Facilities

There are three main types of long-term care homes in Ontario, which as Table 6.1 shows, are operated in the following ways:

- nursing homes are usually operated by private corporations;
- municipal homes for the aged are owned by municipal councils. Many municipalities are required to build a home for the aged in their area, either on their own or in partnership with a neighbouring municipality; and
- charitable homes or not-for-profits, are usually owned by non-profit corporations, such as faith, community, ethnic or cultural groups.

There are several major problems in long-term care facilities in Ontario. The for-profit sector receives government funding for bricks and mortar as well as for services, a situation that has been consistently critiqued by those concerned about the quality of life for seniors as well as by those who are hired to provide care.

The long-term care sector in Ontario is undergoing a significant transformation. There was an addition of almost 20,000 new beds between 2000 and 2007. Most of this expansion has been through the for-profit sector, and this is not likely to change much in the years ahead. At the same time, the provincial government has been eliminating multi-bed wards through upgrades at older long-term care homes across the province. In a July 31, 2007, press release the government announced that there would be 35,000 long-term care beds redeveloped over the next ten years (Ontario Ministry of Health and Long-Term Care 2007). However, the expansion is probably over. The recent focus on developing an Aging at Home Strategy (announced August 28, 2007) signals a policy shift. Many have argued that supportive services in the community are not only what seniors and their families desire, but they are more cost effective. However, the question needs to be asked — cost effective for whom? Aging at home is the *de facto* reality for most older women. It is the quality of their lives that is of concern. What is needed is a policy strategy that ensures that older women, their female kin and paid care providers are supported. A gendered strategy would need to take into consideration the varying social locations of women. The types of supports needed by a frail older woman probably do not map neatly onto what a daughter can provide. The work involved often needs a skill set that requires training—which has costs. Needs and capabilities are both important issues in programming but they cannot be assumed.

## The Future of Long-Term Care in Ontario

There is tremendous variation in the quality of care in Ontario's nursing homes, as anyone connected with the industry knows. Standards, their enforcement and various ways of monitoring them have been suggested by seniors' advocates. Without all three, very vulnerable older people, most of whom are women, continue to be at risk.

In May 2008 yet another two deaths in a Toronto nursing home owned by a for-profit chain led to an inquiry about the quality of care (*Toronto Star* 2008: A1). Not surprisingly, one of the issues highlighted was the shortage of personal support workers (PSWs) — those who provide the hands-on services. Once again residents, as well as PSWs themselves, described working conditions that resulted in aides "being run off their feet." PSW training varies tremendously but at the moment it is basically whatever the hiring agency determines it should be. Thus both residents and personal care workers are put at risk.

The Ontario Health Coalition, a network of over 400 grassroots community organizations committed to enhancing publicly funded, publicly administered health care in the province, has made the development of minimum care standards central to all their public presentations around Bill 140, *The Long-Term Care Act*. Advocates are focusing on the need for staffing standards based on residents' acuity (or required level of care) (OHC 2007). Regulated levels of care were removed by the former Harris government. They are seen as critical for protecting residents and staff from injury, accident and neglect. These would be operationalized into specific hours. Homes at the average level of acuity would be required to provide 3.5 hours of care. Homes above the average would be required to provide care at higher levels and homes below the average would staff at lower levels. Funding is not based directly on individual need but on group average needs in each facility.

Although one can argue with the specifics, staffing standards are fundamental to quality care. Of equal importance is the recommendation that homes prepare a "plan of care" for each resident, outlining the care requirements and levels of service offered. This plan should be reviewed at least every three months and adapted as the resident's needs change. When and if this comes to be, it will be important to monitor whether or not residents have input into their care plan. Women have traditionally been excluded from decisions and control over their own care — without consultation they will continue to be silenced, no matter how good the new standards are.

Long-term care settings need not be the institutions that old and young say they do not want to see themselves or their loved ones in. Some people need more skilled and ongoing care than can be assured in their own homes, or in so-called retirement homes. What if long-term care was thought of as a diverse continuum of housing and care options — with associated standards and monitoring? An aggressive supportive housing policy could offer numerous benefits to aging women and pull Ontario much more in the direction of Sweden with the following kinds of changes:

- Social support would provide an insurance against isolation.
- Care needs would be monitored and services provided and modified accordingly.
- Environments would be gender-sensitive as well as ethno-culturally meaningful and provide residents with a real sense of community
- The benefits to service providers, who are primarily women, would also be profound:
- There would be regulation of working conditions.
- Care would be organized in ways that support care providers rather than monitored as piece work.

Standards take many forms and monitoring occurs in different ways. Community involvement is one way to monitor what is happening in long-term care facilities. Concerned Friends of Ontario Citizens in Care provides some examples of how ethno-cultural communities in Toronto have negotiated spaces to improve the quality of life of their elderly members — spaces that are exclusive and inclusive at the same time (Christensen and Rajzman 2007). For example, the Yee Hong Society has set up several long-term care homes to meet the needs of the Chinese community in the Greater Toronto Area. Using its experience in working with other immigrant communities, Yee Hong in Markham has established a South Asian wing, and in Scarborough-Finch it set aside 25 beds for the local Japanese community. Momiji Health Care Society is a supportive housing complex that serves the Japanese community. Volunteers support staff (e.g., with feeding) in coordination with the workers' union. Seven Oaks Home for the Aged has developed support for Tamil residents and also works with the Armenian community. Armenian residents benefit from the support of community volunteers, who among other things prepare special food and hold community events. After two years of consultations with the Reh'ma Foundation, which serves the Muslim community, Extendicare Scarborough agreed to set aside 12 beds for Muslim residents. The partnership between the Reh'ma Foundation and Extendicare continues, with the foundation providing information about religious practices and appropriate food. Special volunteers are being trained to support the program.

These are promising practices. However, even the most promising reports on long-term care are silent on how gender issues are being addressed. Are these community-based efforts taking into account factors that make women feel at home? These factors will likely be quite different from those that give men a sense of belonging. Such questions need to be raised to ensure that issues of gender equity in health are not eclipsed by homogenizing the needs of impoverished and racialized people along ethno-cultural lines.

Let me conclude by returning to Albert Banerjee's analysis of long-term care in Ontario. If twenty-five years from now long-term care in Ontario has been redesigned with women in mind, I may well be an elderly woman needing intensive chronic care and I may have some cognitive impairment (breakthrough research notwithstanding)—but I will be far less likely to be a depression statistic.

# 7

# What Matters to Women Working in Long-Term Care

## A Union Perspective

Marcy Cohen

The Hospital Employees' Union (HEU) represents more than 90 percent of the staff working in both profit and non-profit licensed residential care facilities across British Columbia. As a result, the HEU has a keen interest in the quality of working and caring conditions in these workplaces. HEU members include licensed practical nurses (LPNs), care aides, activity workers, rehabilitation assistants, dietary and housekeeping staff — everyone except registered nurses (RNs) and rehabilitation/recreation therapists. Ninety percent of the HEU members who work in long-term care are women. Most are between 35 and 50 years old, and many are from immigrant and visible minority backgrounds. In addition, the majority of residents are frail senior women over 80, most of whom are widowed and low-income (Vogal 1999).

The union's role in long-term care dates back to the 1970s, when HEU first organized the staff in the private nursing home sector in B.C. During that organizing drive, the union highlighted issues of resident neglect and low staffing levels, linking poor working conditions for staff with poor caring conditions for residents. The success of this organizing drive and public support for the union's linking of caring and working conditions were critical in pushing the provincial government, in the late 1970s, to establish a legislative and funding framework to improve quality standards in B.C.'s long-term care sector. This included the passage of the 1978 *Long-term Care Act*, the development of funding guidelines for staffing and the provision of financial and expert assistance to support not-for-profit community organizations in building long-term care residential facilities.

Over the years, the union has continued to advocate for improved working and caring conditions. In 2001, based on growing concerns from our members working in long-term care about their capacity to provide appropriate and compassionate care to residents, the union made increased staffing levels a priority bargaining issue. The union worked in coalition with community and seniors' groups to advocate for better staffing levels and negotiated an agreement with the provincial government to add 300 new care aide positions in long-term care.

However, since the election of a Liberal government in May 2001, the union has been on the defensive. In January 2002 the government passed Bill 29, the *Health and Social Services Delivery Improvement Act*, which eliminated negotiated contracting protections for unionized health care workers. Bill 29 resulted in the loss of 9,000 to 10,000 jobs and huge increases in the contracting out and privatization of care and support work (i.e., cleaning, laundry and food services), particularly in long-term care.

In addition, between 2001 and 2004, there was a net closure of 26 publicly funded residential care facilities and the number of residential care beds was reduced by 2,529. Although some assisted living spaces were developed to replace them, there was still a province-wide reduction of 1,464 spaces over the three years (Cohen et al. 2005: 5). Since 2004 a limited number of new long-term care facilities have been built, but almost all have been constructed by private corporations as public-private partnerships.

The evidence points to the problems with this policy shift from residential care to assisted living. For one thing, the vast majority of long-term care residents have dementia and are in need of very complex, personalized care not available within assisted living facilities. In addition, the reduction in long-term care took place at the same time as reductions in home care and hospital services, further adding to the vulnerability of frail seniors (and people with disabilities). As a result, there has been a shift in the burden of care to unpaid caregivers, mostly women, who are now either supporting family members at home or supplementing the care that is provided in assisted living and even in long-term care.

The closure of many long-term care facilities, a shift from not-for-profit to for-profit delivery and the contracting out of health support positions has also had a profound effect on the standards of care in B.C. In many cases, front-line staff report that working and caring conditions have deteriorated with the increase in the number of residents with complex problems and no corresponding rise in staffing levels or training standards. For example, Beacon Hill Villa, a Victoria facility owned by the Retirement Concepts Corporation, contracted out both care and support services following the passage of Bill 29. Since then, health officials have repeatedly cited Beacon Hill for violations of regulations protecting seniors in care, and in 2007 the Health Authority was forced to temporarily take over management of the facility because of the serious nature of the violations.

The potential negative implications of the restructuring of long-term residential care in B.C. is evident in the research. Researchers look at the relationship between both facility ownership and quality of care and work environment and quality of care. They overwhelmingly show not only lower staffing levels and lower quality in private facilities, but also that there is a direct link between worker empowerment and quality of care. And the fact that it is mainly women working in long-term care means that they have been called upon, once again, to make up for staff shortages and lower quality by donating their own unpaid labour to ensure residents do not experience reduced levels of care.

## Lower Quality in For-Profit Care

In 1998, Charlene Harrington, a researcher at the University of California, surveyed data from over 13,000 U.S. long-term care facilities to determine the impact of the profit motive on the quality of care (Harrington 2001: 1453). She showed that there were substantially higher licensing infractions and lower staffing levels in for-profit and chain-operated facilities than in not-for-profit facilities. Profit-making facilities registered 30 percent more standards violations and 41 percent more "severe deficiencies" than non-profit facilities. Chain operations had a particularly bad record: quality-of-care deficiencies (including assessments, infection control and nursing, physician, dietary, rehabilitative, dental and pharmacy services) were 14 percent higher and overall deficiencies 13 percent higher in for-profit chains than in for-profit non-chains (Harrington 2002). In terms of staffing levels, her analysis revealed that nursing hours per patient-day at for-profit facilities were 32 percent lower than at non-profit facilities, and care aide hours were 12 percent lower. Overall staffing, including support services, was 20 percent lower in for-profits than in non-profits. A 2005 overview of the research by University of Toronto professor Michael Hillmer and colleagues recorded similar findings (Hillmer et al. 2005).

Research from British Columbia also indicates lower staffing for both direct care and support staff in for-profit facilities (McGregor et al. 2005). In a study of 76 percent of all B.C. long-term care facilities, the mean number of hours per resident-day was significantly higher — 20 minutes for direct-care staff and 14 minutes for support staff — in the not-for-profit facilities than in the for-profit facilities. The staff in the different facilities had similar wages and benefits determined by a province-wide collective agreement; as a result, the researcher noted, lowering staffing levels was "one of the options available to generate profit" (McGregor et al. 2005).

## The Relationship of Staffing to Quality of Care

A review of the literature (Murphy 2006) includes more than 34 peer review studies looking at the relationship between staffing and quality outcomes for residents. The literature shows that all three levels of care providers — RNs, LPNs and care aides — contribute to quality outcomes. For example, in facilities where licensed staff are available to supervise or assist care aides during mealtimes, the outcomes are significantly better. Other studies examine nurse staffing levels needed to avoid residents suffering from preventable adverse outcomes such as falls, fractures, infections, weight loss, dehydration, pressure ulcers, incontinence, agitated behaviour and hospitalizations. One Canadian study concluded that the ratio of staff to residents in B.C. residential care facilities must be increased, especially on evenings and nights, if aggression is to be prevented (Murphy 2006: 30). Another found that for four of the five measurements, nurse aide staffing below 2.06 hours per resident per day was associated with a quadruple increase in the likelihood of hospitalization (Murphy 2006: 67). There is also a growing recognition that integrating a multi-disciplinary primary care team of physicians and other health professionals into long-term facility care would greatly improve the quality of care.

## Client-Centred Care

In addition to the issue of staffing and ownership, there is also much talk in B.C. as elsewhere about the benefits of moving away from a hierarchical institutional model to a model that focuses on residents' individual abilities and encourages staff to provide individualized support and care. Based on Swedish and Australian models of client-focused or resident-centred care, it was called Gentle Care when first introduced in B.C. in the early 1990s (Gnaedinger 2000). The key elements of the model are "a work culture that values the resident first; flexibility of residents' schedule and care; multi-skilled or multi-tasked front-line care staff; permanent assignments for front-line care staff; care aide/LPN involvement in care planning; respectful management philosophy and practice and small clusters of residents" (Gnaedinger 2000: 4).

However, a HEU-sponsored study of nurses, care aides and other front-line staff in four facilities indicated that effectiveness of the model varied considerably depending on where and how it was implemented. Staff participation in decision-making, the flexible application of the model and adequate staffing were the keys to success. So while most workers were in favour of a client-centred approach they also wanted to have the option to rotate their responsibilities if they found their work with some residents particularly difficult. Others said it did not work well in large institutions or with residents who required particularly heavy physical support (Gnaedinger 2000).

## Safe and Healthy Workplaces Have Higher Staffing Levels

What does in fact make some facilities safer and healthier workplaces than others? The research shows that facilities with low worker injury rates have a combination of higher direct-care staffing levels and a more positive work environment.

A 2003 B.C. study looked at the risk factors for musculoskeletal (MSI) injuries (including sprains and repetitive motion injuries) and aggression-related injuries (including physical abuse such as hitting or kicking and verbal abuse). The study found "significant differences between workloads and work environments in low injury-rate (LIRFs) and high injury-rate facilities (HIRFs)" (Cohen and Yassi 2003: 10). In terms of staffing, high injury-rate facilities had a 16: 1 resident-to-staff ratio, compared to only 12: 1 in low injury-rate facilities, despite similar levels of government funding. Workers in high injury-rate facilities had a greater physical workload and were more negative about their jobs than workers in low injury-rate places, who reported having more supportive and trusting relationships with management, as well as better information-sharing, problem-solving and policy dissemination. The facilities with lower injury rates communicated much more information about the potential aggression of new residents and had fewer aggression-related injuries (24 percent) than those with high injury rates (39 percent).

The study made clear that an engaged environment — which encourages ongoing learning, continuous input from front-line workers and flexibility of care — is key to improving working and caring conditions. It was also important that the workplace had a comprehensive philosophy of care with concrete policies and practices in place to support staff in areas such as resident aggression.

## Empowered Workers Provide More Individualized Care

The relationship between a positive work environment and quality care is further validated in a 2007 B.C. study of 568 formal care providers (RNs, LPNs and care aides). This study examined the relationship between care providers' access to "structural empowerment" and their ability to provide individualized care to residents of long-term care facilities (Boothman 2007). It found that care providers with access to information, support (including access to education and recognition for a job well done), resources and opportunity were more likely to contribute to the provision of high-quality, individualized care. This finding echoes research by Tellis-Nayak (2007), who concluded that when the workplace environment improves quality of life for the care staff, the care staff are increasingly able and willing to add quality of life to the residents.

The quality of relationships in the workplace relates directly to the quality of care providers' work life and the quality of care they provide. Therefore, management needs to address the needs of both care providers and care recipients in order to improve the quality of care in long-term care facilities.

## Making a Difference in Long-Term Facility Care

Many of the issues raised in this chapter — appropriate staffing ratios, profit versus not-for-profit delivery and ensuring effective implementation of an individualized care model — require action at the provincial and/or federal levels, as well as by academics, unions, policy-makers and the public to promote greater collaboration and input from staff and residents on care-related issues. Two of the key mechanisms that can make a difference are mandated advocacy programs and effective oversight and enforcement of licensing requirements in residential care.

The U.S. offers some positive examples of advocacy programs. Since the 1970s, there has been a very strong national consumer movement advocating for residents and staff in long-term care, led by the National Citizens' Coalition for Nursing Home Reform (www.nccnhr.org). This organization was established because of the widely reported problems of abuse, neglect and substandard care in the U.S.'s mainly private long-term care sector. As a result of this advocacy, in 1981 the U.S. government passed the *Older Americans Act*, which mandated, among other things, the Long-Term Ombudsman Program. This program is funded federally and operates in every state. It provides a coordinated approach to advocacy, including a network of locally trained volunteers who advocate on behalf of individual residents and professional staff at the state level.

There is no equivalent in Canada. In B.C., as in other provinces, there are a number of volunteer organizations — including Advocates for Care Reform, the B.C. Coalition to Eliminate Abuse of Seniors and the Seniors Advocacy Network — who advocate on behalf of vulnerable seniors. But there is no federal or provincial legislative mandate or ongoing funding to support the work of these NGOs. In B.C., the Seniors Advocacy Network recently gained support from the Federation of Canadian Municipalities to establish regional seniors' advocacy offices funded by the provincial and federal governments.

In 2004, a report from the Ontario Ministry of Health's Long-Term Care Division recommended that a long-term care ombudsperson be established in Ontario, but this has yet to happen. It is interesting to note that while a number of provinces have ombudsperson programs that act as "watchdogs" for public services, only Nova Scotia has staff whose work focuses specifically on seniors in long-term care. Support from the federal and/or provincial governments for an ombudsperson program for seniors in long-term care is crucial to help tackle the problems in long-term care.

Recent changes in licensing regulations and enforcement in Ontario and Alberta have occurred as a result of extensive media coverage of the substandard care, abuse and neglect in their long-term care facilities. In response to negative media publicity in Ontario in 2004, the Ministry of

Health increased funding for care staff, introduced surprise inspections and a website (http://publicreporting.ltchomes.net) where the public can get information from inspection reports of individual facilities. And in late 2006, they tightened their licensing rules to include improved staff training, whistle-blower protection for staff and residents, 24-hour nursing coverage, a minimum of two baths a week and a resident bill of rights.

In Alberta, the government response to similar negative publicity and an Auditor-General's report that found substandard care in one-third of 25 facilities reviewed, has been slower in coming. The government has announced $42 million to begin in 2009 for increased care staff, but critics argue that will still not bring Alberta's long-term care facilities up to the promised 3.6 hours of care per day.

In B.C., the positive features of the *Community Care and Assisted Living Act* and its regulations include a definition of abuse, whistle-blower protection for staff and residents, mandatory reporting of abuse and mandated abuse-prevention policies. But there are, at the same time, some glaring weaknesses: there are no minimum staffing levels or training requirements, no definition of what should be included in abuse prevention policies, and no public reporting on licensing violations and substantiated complaints. The Ministry of Health's funding formula for long-term care has not been updated since 1979, and access to information on results of complaints investigations and inspections can only be obtained through a Freedom of Information request. There is, in addition, no requirement or dedicated funding for facilities to establish independent family councils and considerable variation among the health authorities in terms of how they implement provincial regulations. These issues require immediate attention to ensure that B.C.'s licensing rules and enforcement mechanisms for long-term care are, in fact, protecting residents from substandard care.

The Hospital Employees Union will continue to focus on improving the quality of care in B.C.'s long-term care facilities, raising the issues of ownership, staffing levels and safe and healthy workplaces as well as the importance of positive relationships between management and staff and staff and residents. In a situation where the majority of the workers and the residents — as well as informal family caregivers — are women, there are numerous shared concerns and countless opportunities for collaboration. Working together to develop and advocate for improvements in quality of care improves the working and living conditions for all of those involved in long-term care.

# 8 Designing Long-Term Care for Lesbian, Gay, Bisexual, Transsexual and Transgender People

Dick Moore

The Homes for the Aged Division in the City of Toronto is working to create a long-term institutional care environment that is safe and comfortable for lesbian, gay, bisexual, transgender and transsexual (LGBTT) women and men. It is a significant initiative and one that merits attention and support. Before I tell you about it, I'd like to give you some background to its development.

I am one of only three people in Canada who is paid to work with older LGBTT people. For many years, my colleague Chris Morrissey — who works at The Centre in Vancouver — and I were the only two. Chris has worked to make home care services more accessible to LGBTT people by training home care workers and providing service education for health care professionals. I have also trained staff working in the home care sector, but most of my work has been in the long-term care sector in city-operated and not-for-profit homes for the aged in Toronto.

There is little Canadian research about long-term care for LGBTT people. A 2006 study that conducted 90 interviews with gay and lesbian seniors, their caregivers and service delivery providers in Quebec, Nova Scotia and British Columbia found that the gays' and lesbians' experiences of homophobia and heterosexism often hampered their ability or willingness to access services and advocate for their needs as seniors. Although most of the service providers interviewed expressed positive intentions towards these clients, their lack of awareness of LGBTT issues "limited their abilities to provide a strong system of support to gay and lesbian seniors" (Brotman, Ryan and Meyer 2006: 2–3).

Our own informal research at the 519 Church Street Community Centre in Toronto has shown similar findings. In 2002, I worked on a Community Sounding Exercise about aging. Many people who participated were concerned about becoming frail and having to depend on home care workers who might neglect or mistreat them because of their sexual orientation or gender identity. LGBTT individuals also expressed their fear of long-term care. Transsexuals especially were wary of poor quality hands-on care. They had heard stories such as that of the nurse who brought other staff into the bathing room to see the "freak," a transsexual woman with a penis.

LGBTT people said they feared that if they needed long-term care, either their needs would not be met or they would have to go back into the closet. One transsexual woman said she would take her life before she would go into long-term care.

An opening for change on behalf of LGBTT seniors was presented by Fudger House, a long-term care home located in the "gaybourhood" of downtown Toronto. Administrator Lorraine Siu was interested in responding to the needs of LGBTT residents in her facility. I took a tour of Fudger House in 2002, and Lorraine and her team expressed interest in supporting their LGBTT residents.

The choice of Fudger House as a place to start was a thoughtful one. It is a city-owned and city-run facility. Staff are represented by a union and the home operates under the City of Toronto's progressive anti-discrimination policy.

As a first step, I worked with the Fudger House management team to plan and implement a staff training program on LGBTT cultural awareness. It is the equivalent of a "101" course, providing participants with basic vocabulary and then exploring the myths and stereotypes about gay people and debunking them.

In October 2006 Sandra Pitters, Director of the Homes for the Aged Division of the City of Toronto, decided to undertake an LGBTT initiative to provide a safe, positive environment in long-term care for its queer residents. She recruited a Steering Committee that included senior divisional staff and representatives from the Community Care Access Centre (which places frail elders in long-term care), the Local Health Integration Network (the Ontario equivalent of a Regional Health Authority), allies from community agencies, lawyers and representatives of resident and family councils.

The following thirteen objectives for the LGBTT initiative were laid out:

- provide leadership, support and encouragement in implementing gay-positive services;
- promote full and equal access to services for LGBTT individuals needing long-term care;
- create an atmosphere of openness and affirmation;
- create an environment where it is safe to be "out";
- offer support for LGBTT residents, their partners and families;
- plan, develop, coordinate and implement care and service protocols that respect LGBTT culture, traditions and social networks;

- plan, develop, coordinate and implement administrative practices that facilitate demonstration of gay-positive care and service;
- build a volunteer program with connections to the LGBTT community.
- develop linkages for LGBTT referrals;
- develop processes to maintain community engagement;
- develop gay-straight alliances of interested residents, their partners, families and staff to provide advice and input to the creation of a gay-positive environment, LGBTT programming and quality improvement.
- research, develop and provide staff training for cultural competence in dealing with LGBTT residents; and
- develop indicators to evaluate LGBTT services.

The Steering Committee was divided into six work groups to deal with different aspects of this organizational change process: Welcoming Environment, Administrative Practices, Programming, Health Care, Human Resources and Community Engagement.

The Welcoming Environment work group was set up to develop some quick initiatives that would give the process focus and momentum. It published a brochure for families that includes the information on the LGBTT initiative, including the following:

- a statement indicating that the homes welcome all citizens of Toronto requiring long-term care, including LGBTT citizens;
- a notice that residents of the home will be meeting and living with residents who identify as LGBTT;
- some residents may be sharing a room, a table in the dining room and daily activities with residents who identify as LGBTT;
- family members of straight residents may identify as LGBTT and may be members of various committees (e.g., family council); and
- a recommendation to hold Pride events in homes, including displays in lobbies (providing archival resources and websites), and to participate in the Pride parade and hold Pride dances.

The Welcoming Environment group advocated for a buddy system for new LGBTT residents and the "judicious" use of rainbow stickers on office doors of supportive staff to indicate gay friendliness. It also promoted the display of the anti-discrimination statement, "We serve all people of Toronto, including LGBTT." It encouraged the inclusion of images of gay and lesbian couples in pictures that decorate the home and in promotion and publicity material, the development of a manual of resource material for staff and volunteers, and the holding of information sessions on LGBTT issues for residents and their families.

The Administrative Practices work group reviewed all the forms used by the homes administration to ensure they used appropriate language regarding sexual orientation and gender identity. It suggested changes to some categories, such as replacing "marital status" with "partnership status" and including "neither" or "both" along with "male" and "female" in the gender category.

The Programming work group had an ambitious agenda. It was chaired by the Manager of Programs and Services (a senior staff position) in one of the homes designated as LGBTT-friendly, and involved residents, staff, chaplains, family members and volunteers. This work group developed a template for a long-term care facility-based Gay-Straight Alliance. It reviewed recreation, dining, social activities and social support programs, spiritual and religious care to see how they could better accommodate LGBTT residents.

The Programming work group established LGBTT-specific programs, including a film night, a book club, a library, a discussion group, an excursion group and various Pride program initiatives. Members developed a workshop on specialty programming for LGBTT residents and programming for mixed groups of residents. The mixed group programming integrates LGBTT issues and concerns into otherwise generic programs and activities (e.g., mentioning a film star who lived a closeted life for fear of being sidelined if it were known s/he was LGBTT).

The chaplaincy aspect of the Programming work group agenda has involved developing a group for family members who are opposed to the LGBTT initiative where they have a chance to be heard and educated.

The Health Care work group worked to ensure that intake and health care would be LGBTT-friendly and sensitive. This work group considered a number of issues involved in providing hands-on care, including:

- the initial assessment process and how it affects LGBTT residents, their partners, families and friends;
- ways of asking questions that are open, sensitive and promote a sense of safety to LGBTT residents, their partners, families and friends; and
- the need for staff training and access to information prior to and during the assessment that can lead to a better understanding of the residents' needs, strengths and desires.

The Health Care work group developed a draft "companion document" for health care workers to increase their sensitivity and knowledge in working with LGBTT seniors. This document highlighted the issue of hands-on care for transsexual residents and the need for orientation and training of nursing and personal care staff.

The Human Resources work group was responsible for reviewing the recruitment, orientation, continuing education and training of staff and volunteers as well as the Family Committee, Home Advisory Committee and Residents' Council. It aimed to ensure the development and maintenance of an inclusive, non-discriminatory workplace environment for gay, lesbian, bisexual and transgender employees, volunteers and residents. This involved developing written policies that include but are not limited to non-discrimination, diversity and non-harassment policies that explicitly include gay, lesbian, bisexual and transgender employees. Its activities included the following:

- active recruitment in the LGBTT community using queer-friendly job boards, e-lists and websites;
- development and implementation or revision of existing policies to ensure effective procedures for dealing with employee complaints of discrimination or harassment based on sexual orientation or gender identity;
- written notice to all employees that discrimination or harassment of other employees on the basis of sexual orientation or gender identification is grounds for appropriate levels of discipline, up to and including dismissal; and
- acquiring and developing resources for staff and volunteer training and continuing education.

The Centre for Addiction and Mental Health was contracted to hold a two-day workshop, "Asking the Right Questions," to train intake workers, social workers, counsellors and others to talk with clients about sexual orientation and gender identity.

The Community Engagement work group determined how to collaborate with the LGBTT community and how to keep residents connected to their community. It developed recommendations regarding community outreach and what we called in-reach.

The outreach aspect was concerned with finding out about and making contact with LGBTT organizations and agencies in the community. It sought ways to collaborate, recruit volunteers and benefactors, and develop and maintain residents' linkages with these groups — using the gay media to advertise the welcoming activities of the home, its various activities and the need for LGBTT volunteers.

Outreach also involved the Community Care Access Centre (CCAC), the organization responsible for placing people in the home, as well as hospital discharge planners, other homes for the aged and retirement homes. The interview and assessment process used by the CCAC and mandated by the Ministry of Health and Long-Term Care fails even to mention, much less address, the matter of sexual orientation or gender identity. Unfortunately, the CCAC was unable to make any changes to the assessment process.

The in-reach efforts involved internal stakeholders such as staff and volunteers, the residents' council, family committee and home advisory committee, whose ideas and suggestions were solicited right from the beginning of the welcoming initiative. It also recommended recruiting LGBTT residents to be buddies of new residents and for leadership roles on the residents' council and the Gay-Straight Alliance, and recruiting LGBTT family members and family members of LGBTT residents to serve on family committees.

Where do we go from here? The Steering Committee plans to develop a report and toolkit with examples of policies, procedures and resource materials for use in other long-term care facilities that want to become LGBTT-safe and LGBTT-friendly. The Steering Committee has developed a relationship with Dr. Shari Brotman of the Faculty of Social Work at McGill University, who has agreed to do an evaluation of the initiative. The first phase of this evaluation is an interview process of all involved as Steering Committee members and a documentation of the process.

What I've learned from this experience of organizational change is that leadership needs to come from a variety of locations within a home. The administrator and management staff are key players and it is critical that they "buy in" to the process. Residents themselves and family members also play a critical role. In one home, a champion of the initiative was appointed to facilitate the various stages of the process. This appointment of an openly gay senior manager has been especially successful. Where such a champion has not been appointed, progress has lagged. Leadership at all levels must be consistent and make a strong commitment of time and resources.

Finally, we should commend the Homes for the Aged Division of the City of Toronto for undertaking this initiative. It started with Fudger House and has been implemented in two of the other nine Toronto homes. Each home has had a different experience, reflecting its location, the comfort of staff in being "out," the commitment of the local management team and the presence of "out" residents and family members.

A final note for consideration or speculation is the need for long-term care facilities specifically designed and built for the LGBTT community and its allies. Certainly the numbers in Toronto and other large urban areas in North America indicate there is a sufficient population base to justify such developments. Numerous ethnic and religious communities have organized and raised funds to build facilities for their members.

There have been occasional, short-term efforts to develop a long-term care home for Toronto's LGBTT community. Most have faltered when the organizers encountered roadblocks. Pride House, an effort of several gay men, has been unable to attract capital funds and buy-in to a particular fundraising initiative. Croneland, a rural lesbian community, was a going concern with a website and plans for different types of buildings that would accommodate women at various stages of wellness. It fell by the wayside when its leader moved away. Other efforts have stalled when the leadership moved on to other projects, got sick, moved away or died.

The amounts involved in terms of fundraising are significant and require high-level leadership, expertise in government relations and knowledge of rules and regulations governing such facilities. The effort requires leadership that will be there for the long run, as well as younger people who see the need and are dedicated to the project's ultimate success. Political leadership on the part of government will also be required. Although the gay liberation movement has come a long way, it is foreseeable that the religious right will vocally oppose the allocation of government funding for such a facility.

It remains my conviction that all long-term care facilities should be safe and comfortable places for LGBTT residents, whether they are public institutions, religiously affiliated or ethnically based. Our human rights code demands it. Sadly, we have a long way to go before we will see such developments.

# 9

# Are There Lessons to Learn from Sweden?

Marta Szebehely

A large European survey asked the following question of a representative sample of the population in 25 countries: "Let's suppose you had an elderly father or mother who lived alone. What do you think would be best if this parent could no longer manage to live on his/her own?"

In Greece, 89 percent of the respondents answered that they would prefer to live together with or to move closer to their parent and 11 percent answered that the parent should stay at home and receive health care and other services in the home. Only 0.4 percent suggested that the parent should move to an old people's home or a nursing home. In contrast, only 16 percent of Swedish respondents suggested that living together or closer to each other would be the best solution, while 41 percent preferred home-based care services and 43 percent argued that residential care would be the best option. Greece and Sweden are two extremes with regard to residential care. Overall, in the 25 countries in the extended European Union, 11 percent said they preferred a nursing home or an old people's home for a parent who could not manage on his or her own (Alber and Köhler 2004: 75).

Do these figures suggest that Swedish elderly people are abandoned by their children? Or do they indicate that there are national differences in how residential care is perceived by the general pubic, differences which in turn are related to differences in access to and quality of residential care? Without going into detail on Greek eldercare, I argue that the latter interpretation is closer to the truth. I contend that the frail elderly in Sweden today generally do find residential care facilities fairly decent places to live — and to die — in.

This conclusion is also suggested by the authors of the European survey report:

> Family solidarity may be just as strong in Sweden as elsewhere in Europe, but the quality of residential care may be so much higher that people have comparatively high trust in state provided solutions and hence little reservation about leaving their parents with the

> support of high-quality public services including residential care facilities. (Alber and Köhler 2004: 74)

The strong support for residential care in Sweden reflected in the survey was also evident during the 2006 Swedish election. The shortage of places in residential care was clearly articulated by the elderly and became a heated political issue during the election campaign. Elderly individuals and representatives of seniors' organizations expressed their fear of not being able to move to residential care when needed. In Sweden today there is a political consensus of the need to halt the closing of institutions and to build new facilities for old people who need more care and support than they can get in their homes.

So if older people in Sweden have more positive attitudes towards residential care than older people in many other countries, what is the explanation? What is residential care in the Swedish context?

## Resources for Eldercare Services: Sweden and Canada

Sweden is the most generous country in the OECD when it comes to public spending on eldercare services: it spends 2.74 percent of its GDP compared to 0.99 percent on average in the OECD and in Canada (OECD 2005: 26). Sweden also has the world's oldest population: 5 percent are 80 years and older compared to 3 percent in Canada (OECD 2005: 101). If we take into account the different proportions of old people in the population in different countries, Sweden spends 71 percent more than the OECD average while Canadian spending on care services for older people is only 3 percent above the OECD average (calculated from OECD 2005: 26, 101).

"Aging in place" and "de-institutionalization" — attempts to shift resources from residential to home-based care — have, for some decades, been the principles underpinning eldercare policies in most Western countries. However, in most (if not all) countries, the bulk of public money spent on eldercare goes to residential care: 72 percent in Sweden and 83 percent in Canada (OECD 2005: 26). Public spending on residential care in Sweden is 58 percent above the OECD average, while in Canada it is 33 percent above the average (OECD 2005: 26). If we can trust the OECD statistics, public spending on residential care is clearly above the average in both Sweden and Canada — in Sweden as a result of more generous spending on eldercare in general, in Canada as a result of resources being more strongly directed to residential care than to home-based care services than in most OECD countries.

Another difference between Sweden and Canada is the role of private spending in residential care. In Sweden 95 percent of the total financial resources for residential care comes from taxes, compared to 77 percent in Canada (calculated from OECD 2005: 26). Hence the individual elderly user bears a larger share of the costs in Canada than in Sweden.

Finally, the division between public and private provision of services differs between the two countries. In Canada almost half of residents live in facilities run by for-profit companies, about one-quarter in not-for-profit facilities and another quarter in facilities run by the government sector (Statistics Canada 2007c, table 3). In Sweden, the vast majority of eldercare services is publicly provided. In both countries, however, there is an increase of private, for-profit providers. In Sweden this increase started in the early 1990s. Non-public providers of publicly financed eldercare services expanded in the 1990s, from less than 3 percent in 1993 to 13 percent in 2000 — 3 percent in not-for-profit organizations and 10 percent in profit-seeking companies, mostly large international firms (Trydegård 2003). Compared to Canada, however, private sector involvement in eldercare in Sweden is still comparatively small.

## Residential Care and Other Care Services in Sweden

Although the majority of public eldercare resources are spent on residential care, other forms of care services cover much larger numbers of elderly people. In 2005, of the 1.7 million elderly people in Sweden (65 years and older), 100,000 lived in residential care. At the same time 135,000 received home care services in their own homes, 300,000 were eligible for subsidized transportation services in taxis or specially adapted vehicles, 160,000 had a personal safety alarm, 65,000 received a home adaptation grant and 20,000 used short-term residential care or day care (SALAR 2007).

Compared to the OECD average, the coverage of care services to Swedish older people is relatively high (OECD 2005), but there has been a drastic decline in both home care services and residential care over the last two to three decades. In 1980, 28 percent of the elderly (80 plus) lived in residential care, compared to only 16 percent today. The decrease in residential care has not been followed by an increase in the number of older people receiving home help. On the contrary, the proportion of elders 80 years and older in the population who receive publicly financed home help decreased from 34 percent to 21 percent during the same period (Szebehely 2005a; NBHW 2007a). As a consequence of this decline, there has been an increase in informal care, which is provided mainly by spouses and daughters of the elderly. Survey studies show that the majority of older people in Sweden prefer public services to family help. Yet the number of elderly women who receive help from their daughters and other family members is far greater than the number who said they preferred to have such help. For instance, among older women who need help with personal care such as bathing, only 7 percent prefer to be helped by a daughter or other relatives but 29 percent actually get help with bathing from their daughters (Szebehely 2005b: 165). The offloading to family care is thus unwanted from the perspective of elderly people themselves. This "informalization" of care is also in contradiction with Swedish family legislation and eldercare policies stating that it is the municipality — not children or other family members — that is responsible for providing care for elderly people, according to need.

The cutbacks of Swedish eldercare services have affected women's everyday lives more than men's. The majority (70 percent) of elderly people who live in residential care or who receive home care services are women (NBHW 2007a). This is mainly a consequence of the fact that old women in general live longer but are sicker and frailer than men. Women usually outlive their husbands — seven out of ten men are married when they die compared to one out of four women (Szebehely 2005b). Most often, older men receive the care they need from their wives while older women, who probably end their life as widows, usually become a home care recipient or a resident in a residential care facility during their lifetime.

Wives and daughters are the most frequent informal carers, and according to Swedish survey data, two-thirds of all informal care for elderly and disabled people is provided by women (Szebehely 2005b). Formal care is even more unevenly distributed between men and women: 95 percent of the Swedish eldercare workers are women (NBHW 2008). Care — paid as well as unpaid — is thus a highly gendered issue in Sweden as in other countries.

In recent years, there is an increased awareness in Swedish policy of the consequences for women of eldercare restructuring. Since 2002, the National Board of Health and Welfare has been commissioned by the Swedish government to regularly review health care and social services from a gender equality perspective. In a recent report gender issues are discussed from the point of view of all three parties involved: the staff, frail elderly people and their family members. The importance of recruiting more men as care workers is stressed. The Board also argues that the development of accessibility and quality of public eldercare services has an impact on gender equality in the general society and affects women both as care recipients and as family members of elderly persons in need of care. The Board concludes:

> There is a risk that the development in recent years with fewer places in residential care and an increasing number of older people living in their ordinary dwellings will shift the responsibility even more towards family members. There is a high risk that this will hit elderly people's children and especially the daughters, i.e., women who already provide the majority of unpaid domestic work. Eldercare services have an important role for gender equality in the entire society. (NBHW 2008: 73)

For elderly persons who do receive public home help, the average number of hours has increased. Help is provided with household chores as well as with personal care. Most home care recipients receive five hours per week or less, but there is no formal upper limit on the number of hours, and some older persons receive help around the clock, six to eight times a day (SALAR 2007).

All forms of care services (including nursing homes and other forms of residential care but not health care) are covered by the *Social Services Act*. According to the Act, everybody who needs help to support themselves has the right to claim assistance from the municipality. An elderly person in need of home care or a place in a nursing home or other forms of residential care has a statutory right to claim service and care and to have his or her needs assessed by turning to the municipality through a single-entry system (the same for residential and home-based care services). The needs assessment is carried out by a municipal care manager, usually a social worker. A person who is not satisfied with the decision can appeal it to an administrative court (Ministry of Health and Social Affairs 2007).

Not only is the legislation and the entry point to services the same for residential and home-based care services in Sweden, the user fees are also set in the same way. No services are means tested, but the user fee is related to income and the amount of help. A max-fee reform in 2002 capped the fees in home care as well as in residential care to SEK 1,620 per month (CAD$ 273). Persons with low incomes may be exempted from paying fees — in 2005 about 30 percent did not pay any fee at all (SALAR 2007). Low-income elderly persons are eligible for a state-financed housing allowance that covers up to 93 percent of their cost for housing or in exceptional cases the entire cost — in their ordinary housing as well as in residential care (Swedish Social Insurance Agency 2008). There is therefore no major economic incentive for an older individual either to move to or to refrain from moving to residential care.

In accordance with the universal Swedish welfare model, following a needs assessment, the same kind of residential care facilities and other services are offered to and used by all social groups. Thus with very few exceptions (a small number of fully privately financed facilities) rich and poor older persons live in the same facilities. There is no possibility of "topping up"; a better-off older person is not allowed to pay extra money and get better services in residential care.

## What Does Swedish Residential Care Look Like?

Despite the de-institutionalization trend in Sweden and the wide range of home-based care services, residential care is still an important alternative for the frailest elderly, especially for single-living elderly with dementia.

In Sweden since 1992, only one concept for residential care is used in legislation and statistics: "special housing," which covers what was formerly known as nursing homes, as well as all other publicly subsidized and needs-assessed combinations of accommodation and care (e.g., old-age homes, group homes for persons with dementia and assisted living).

The year 1992 was an important turning point, when the responsibility for nursing homes was shifted from the health care sector in the county councils to the municipal sector and social services. Since then all forms of residential care are regarded as social care rather than health care, and the housing standard, including the individual's right to privacy, has improved radically. The elderly person is now formally regarded as a tenant and rent is paid separately from the fee for care and services.

Before the 1980s a Swedish nursing home often looked like a hospital, with large buildings and shared bedrooms. There are still some larger facilities of this type, but on average there are 32 residents in a residential care facility in Sweden today. One-fifth of residents live in small units with ten places or fewer for persons with dementia (NBHW 2007b). Even in a large facility, not more than ten people usually live on the same floor. Meals are generally served in a combined kitchen and dining-room on the floor rather than in a large common dining-hall.

Today almost all older people in residential care have their own private room or small apartment. Private furniture (usually with the exception of the bed) is the rule. Only 2 percent of the elderly in residential care share their room/apartment with another person (other than a spouse). More than 90 percent of residents also have a private bathroom, and more than 70 percent have private cooking facilities, usually a kitchenette (NBHW 2007a). Although the cooking facilities are rarely used by residents, who are often too frail to do housework, visiting relatives and friends may use the stove to prepare a meal or coffee for themselves and the resident.

Hence, since 1992, the principles of Swedish residential care have been guided by a "social" model, with a norm of small care units and a relatively high degree of privacy. The care workers are "generalists": that is, they provide all kinds of help — including care of the body and of the environment — for a limited numbers of residents. There is usually no specialized cleaning, laundry or housekeeping staff, and in the small facilities that dominate the sector, there is usually no specialized staff for recreation and other activities, and sometimes no kitchen staff.

It is actually part of official Swedish residential care ideology, especially in smaller units for elderly persons with dementia, for residents and care workers to prepare meals and do other household activities together. This is not always the case, but it is not unusual. In response to concerns about hygiene, the National Board of Health and Welfare recently published recommendations in this area. The Board affirmed that residents are allowed to spend time in the kitchen and to participate in cooking. It stresses that staff need to be trained about risks in handling food, but the underlying message is that normal caution is enough: both staff and residents should wash their hands, use an apron and not deal with food if they have any infectious disease (NBHW 2007c).

Compared to Sweden, Canadian residential care facilities are larger and more hospital-like in terms of architecture and organization of the care work (Eales et al 2001; Armstrong and Banerjee: chapter 1 in this volume). Canadian residential care facilities have an average of 96 places and 70 percent of the residents live in facilities with more than 100 beds (Statistics Canada 2007c: 11, 18).

From a Canadian perspective "the Swedish model" has been described as "resident centred" and characterized by "small clusters of residents," with "flexibility of residents' schedule and care; multi-skilled or multi-tasked workers; permanent assignments for front line staff (little or no rotation); front line workers' involvement in care planning" (Gnaedinger 2003: 358). Gnaedinger discusses some attempts to move Canadian dementia care from a "medical and hierarchical model, which stresses residents' incapacities and staff's obligation to follow rigid schedules, to a social model, which emphasizes each resident's individuality and abilities, and empowers staff to flexibly provide support and care" (Gnaedinger 2003: 358). The implementation of the new model was only partly successful. Interviews with care workers showed that they were usually positive towards it, but they noted several barriers to implementing it in their workplaces, such as low staffing levels, high workload and "the large scale and hospital-like design of the typical long-term care facility in Canada." It was not possible to simply import a new ideology of care to a setting very different in terms of resources, physical environment and hierarchies (Gnaedinger 2003; see also Beattie 1998; Keating et al. 2001).

When the care workers in Gnaedinger's study were asked to describe an ideal facility for elderly people with dementia, they described an environment quite different from the places they were working. In their visions, it should "look like a house," there should be no more than ten residents per unit or eating together in one dining-room, and the residents should have personalized, private bedrooms with private bathrooms. The staff-to-resident ratio would be 1: 4 or 1: 5, and the residents' days would be flexible and have meaningful activities.

## Lessons Learned from Sweden

Swedish residential care is certainly not without problems. One problem is the recent dramatic reduction of places in residential care (NBHW 2007d). An overview of the quality in residential care facilities by the National Board of Health and Welfare points at a shortage of trained staff, high proportions of part-time and casual employees (which negatively affects the continuity of care), lack of choice in terms of meals, too much time between dinner and breakfast (the evening meal is often served too early) and large differences in these respects as well as in staffing levels between municipalities (NBHW 2007b). Both the Board and independent researchers have pointed at boredom and a lack of social activities in residential care. Other areas of critique are that persons with dementia are sometimes living with other older persons or persons with psychiatric disorders.

Compared to many other countries, however, the quality of Swedish residential care is high. The visions expressed by the care workers in Gnaedinger's study are much closer to a typical Swedish than a typical Canadian residential care facility. Gnaedinger shows that it is not easy to move care models from one context to another. But with this in mind, it is still possible to learn some lessons from Swedish residential care and from the comparison between Canadian and Swedish eldercare:

- *Resources matter*. An appropriate staffing ratio is probably the single most important condition for quality care.
- *Architecture matters*. It is easier to provide good care in a small facility, and a good residential care facility should have spaces for both privacy *and* togetherness.
- *Ideologies of care matter*. A hospital is not a good role model for care of people who most probably will not recover from their illnesses but rather become more and more frail over time. A social perspective on aging is important even when residents have large medical needs. Good residential care combines safety *and* independence.
- *Organization of care work matters*. A hierarchical organization with predetermined occupational tasks and detailed regulations is an obstacle to good care. In order to provide good care there has to be enough *time* and *continuity* in the encounters between the care worker and the resident, a *limited number of residents* for each worker to relate to and sufficient *freedom of action* for the worker to adapt to the different and changing situations of the care recipients.
- *Gender matters*. If residential care is not accessible or not good enough, it is women in particular who are affected: frail older women who need residential care, their daughters and other family members, as well as the care workers. Therefore all changes in residential care and other eldercare services need to be reviewed from a gender perspective.
- *Residential care is not enough*. A wide range of high-quality support and facilities are essential if family members — in practice mainly women — are not to end up providing care, disregarding their own needs. Informal care can only be voluntary if there are good formal alternatives.

# Bibliography

Alber, J. and U. Köhler. 2004. *Health and Care in an Enlarged Europe*. Quality of Life in Europe. Dublin: European Foundation for the Improvement of Living and Working Conditions.

Alberta Health and Wellness. 2006. Annual Report. http://www.health.alberta.ca/newsroom/annual-report-2007.html

_____. 2004. *Advancing the Mental Health Agenda: A Provincial Mental Health Plan for Alberta*. Provincial Mental Health Planning Project. Edmonton, AB: Alberta Health and Wellness.

_____. 2000. *Strategic Directions and Future Actions: Healthy Aging and Continuing Care in Alberta*. Edmonton, Alberta. http://www.assembly.ab.ca/lao/library/egovdocs/alhw/2000/128094.pdf.

Alberta Mental Health Board. 2006. A Framework for Alberta, "Healthy Aboriginal People in Healthy Communities." http://www.amhb.ab.ca/publications.

Assembly of First Nations (AFN). 2005 "First Nations Action Plan on Continuing Care." Ottawa, Ontario.

Alexander, Taylor. 2002. "The History and Evolution of Long-Term Care in Canada." In Marion Stephenson and Eleanor Sawyer, eds., *Continuing the Care: The Issues and Challenges for Long-Term Care*. Ottawa, ON: CHA Press.

Armstrong, Pat, with Albert Banerjee. 2007. "Challenging Questions: Designing Long-Term Facility Care with Women in Mind." Toronto: Women and Health Care Reform Group (Draft).

Armstrong, Pat, Hugh Armstrong and Krista Scott-Dixon. February 2006. *Critical to Care: Women and Ancillary Work in Health Care*. Available from The National Coordinating Group on Health Care Reform and Women (http://www.ce-whcesf. ca/healthreform/).

Armstrong, Pat, and Tamara Daly. 2004. *"There Are Not Enough Hands": Conditions in Ontario's Long-Term Care Facilities*. Report prepared for the Canadian Union of Public Employees. Toronto.

Armstrong, Pat, and Irene Jansen, with Mavis Jones and Erin Connell. 2003. "Assessing the Impact of Restructuring and Work Reorganization in Long-Term Care." In Penny Van Esterik, ed., *Head, Heart and Hand Partnerships for Women's Health in Canadian Environments* Vol. 1. Toronto: National Network on Environments and Women's Health. http://www.yorku.ca/nnewh.

Armstrong, Pat, and Olga Kitts. 2004. "Caregiving in Historical Perspective." In Paul Leduc Browne, ed., *The Commodity of Care: Assessing Ontario's Experiment with Managed Competition in Home Care*. Ottawa: Canadian Centre for Policy Alternatives.

Armstrong, Pat, and Kate Laxer. 2006. "Precarious Employment, Privatization, and the Health-Care Industry: The Case of Ancillary Workers." In Leah Vosko, ed., *Precarious Employment: Understanding Labour Market Insecurity in Canada*. Kingston:

McGill-Queen's University Press.

Baines, Donna. 2004. "Caring for Nothing. Work Organization and Unwaged Labour in Social Services." *Work, Employment and Society* 18(2): 267–95.

Bartels, S., K. Levine and D. Shea. 1999. "Community Based Long-Term Care for Older Persons with Severe and Persistent Mental Illness in an Era of Managed Care." *Psychiatric Services* 50(9): 1189–97.

Beattie, W. 1998. "Current Challenges to Providing Personalized Care in a Long Term Care Facility." *Leadership in Health Services* 11(2).

Bent, Kathy. 2004. "Anishinaabe Ik-We Mino-Aie-Win. Aboriginal Women's Health Issues: A Holistic Perspective on Wellness." University of Athabasca.

Bernstein, M.A., and R. Hensley. 1993. "Developing Community-Based Program Alternatives for the Seriously and Persistently Mentally Ill Elderly." *Journal of Mental Health Administration* 20: 201–207.

Berta, Whitney, Audrey Laporte, Dara Zarnett, Vivian Valdmanis and Geoffrey Anderson. 2006. "A Pan-Canadian Perspective on Institutional Long-Term Care." *Health Policy* 79: 175–94.

Boothman, Sienna. 2007. "The Influence of Care Provider Access to Structural Empowerment on Individualized Care in Long Term Care Facilities." MA Thesis, Dept. of Gerontology, Simon Fraser University.

Brant, Clare. 1994. "Native Issues." In R. Grant, ed., *Images in Psychiatry*. World Psychiatric Association, Canada.

Brotman, Shari, Bill Ryan and Elizabeth Meyer. March 2006. "The Health and Social Service Needs of Gay and Lesbian Seniors and Their Families in Canada." Montreal: McGill School of Social Work. Canadian Institutes of Health Research, Social Science and Humanities Research Council of Canada. CSSS Cavendish/University Affiliated Research Centre in Social Gerontology. http://www.mcgill.ca/files/interaction/Executive_Summary.pdf.

Browne, A., and V. Smye 2002. "A Postcolonial Analysis of Health Care Discourses Addressing Aboriginal Women." *Nurse Researcher* 9(3): 28–37.

Buchignani, N., and C. Armstrong-Esther. 1999. Informal Care and Older Native Canadians. *Aging and Society* 19: 3–32.

Caro, Francis. 2006. "Family and Aging Policy." *Journal of Aging and Social Policy* 18(3/4): 1–5.

Castle, Nicholas, Steven Handler, John Engberg and Kristen Sonon. 2007. "Nursing Home Administrators' Opinions of the Resident Safety Culture in Nursing Homes." *Health Care Management Review* 32(1): 66–764.

Christensen, Joan, and Ellen Rajzman. 2007. *Creating Welcoming Communities in Long-Term Care Homes: Support for Ethno-cultural and Spiritual Diversity*. A Project of Concerned Friends of Ontario Citizens in Care Facilities. Christensen Community Consulting.

CIHI (Canadian Institute for Health Information). 2006. "Facility-Based Continuing Care in Canada 2004–2005." Ottawa: Canadian Institute for Health Information.

Cloutier-Fisher, Denise, and Mark W. Skinner. 2006. "Leveling the Playing Field? Exploring the Implications of Managed Competition for Voluntary Sector Providers of Long-term Care in Small Town Ontario." *Health and Place* 12: 97–109.

CMHC (Canada Mortgage and Housing Corporation). 2007. *Retirement Homes Report* — *Ontario.* http://www.cmhc-schl.gc.ca/odpub/esub/64651/64651_2007_A01.pdf.

Cohen, Marcy. October 2006. "Union Perspectives on Abuse Prevention in Long-Term Care: Current Situation, Future Possibilities." Unpublished paper.

Cohen, Marcy, Janice Murphy, Kelsey Nutland and Aleck Ostry. 2005. *Continuing Care: Renewal or Retreat? BC Residential and Home Health Care Restructuring 2001-2004.* Vancouver: Canadian Centre for Policy Alternatives BC Office.

Cohen, Marcy, and Annalee Yassi. 2003. *Reducing Injuries in Intermediate Care: Risk Factors for Musculoskeletal and Violence-related Injuries Among Care Aides and Licensed Practical Nurses in Intermediate Care Facilities.* A joint project of WCB, HEU, Occupational Health and Safety Agency for Healthcare in BC, Institute of Health Promotion Research, Canadian Institutes of Health Research, University of British Columbia. February.

Coster, A. Hinds, and J. Bodnarchuk. 2006. "Using Administrative Data to Develop Indicators of Quality of Care in Personal Care Homes." Winnipeg: Manitoba Centre for Health Policy.

Coughlan, Rory, and Linda Ward. 2007. "Experiences of Recently Relocated Residents of Long-Term Care Facility in Ontario: Assessing Quality Qualitatively." *International Journal of Nursing Studies* 44: 47–57.

Department of Health, Nova Scotia. 2007. "Continuing Care." In *Nova Scotia Department of Health, Continuing Care Branch*: Nova Scotia Department of Health, Continuing Care Branch. http://www.gov.ns.ca/health/ccs/default.htm.

Doupe, M., M. Brownell, A. Kozyrskyj, N. Dik, C. Burchill, M. Dahl, D. Chateau, C. De Dumont-Smith. 2002. *Aboriginal Elder Abuse in Canada.* http://www.ahf.ca/pages/download/28_37.

Doupe, M., M. Brownell, A. Kozyrskyj, N. Dik, C. Burchill, M. Dahl, D. Chateau, C. DeCoster, A. Hinds and J. Bodnarchuk. 2006. *Using Administrative Data to Develop Indicators of Quality of Care in Personal Care Homes.* Winnipeg: Manitoba Centre for Health Policy.

Dumont-Smith, Claudette. 2002. *Aboriginal Elder Abuse in Canada.* http://www.ahf.ca/pages/download/28_37.

Eales, J., N. Keating and A. Damsma. 2001. "Seniors' Experiences of Client-centred Residential Care." *Ageing and Society* 21: 279–96.

FNIH (First Nations and Inuit Health). 2007. "Statistical Profile on the Health of First Nations in Canada." First Nations and Inuit Health. http://www.hc-sc.gc.ca/fnih-spni/pubs/gen/stats_profil_e.html.

Fuller, S., C. Fuller and M. Cohen. 2003. *Health Care Restructuring in BC: A CCPA Policy Brief.* Vancouver: Canadian Centre for Policy Alternatives, BC Office.

Gass, Thomas Edward. 2004. *Nobody's Home: Candid Reflections of a Nursing Home Aide.* Ithaca: Cornell University Press.

Gee, E.M., and G.M. Gutman. 2000. *The Overselling of Population Aging: Apocalyptic Demography, Intergenerational Challenges and Social Policy.* Don Mills, ON: Oxford Press.

Gnaedinger, Nancy. 2003. "Changes in Long-Term Care for Elderly People with Dementia: A Report from the Front Lines in British Columbia, Canada." In A. Weiner and J. Ronch, eds., *Culture Change in Long-Term Care.* New York: Haworth Press.

_____. 2000. *Changes in Long Term Care for Elderly People with Dementia: A Report from the Front Lines*. Vancouver: Hospital Employees' Union of BC. September 4.

Grant, Karen, et al., eds. 2004. *Caring For/Caring About: Women, Home Care and Unpaid Caregiving*. Aurora, ON: Garamond.

Guberman, Nancy. 2004. "Designing Home and Community Care for the Future: Who Needs Care?" In Karen Grant, et al. *Caring For/Caring About: Women, Home Care and Unpaid Caregiving*. Aurora, ON: Garamond.

Guberman, Nancy, Jean-Pierre Lavoie, Michel Fournier, Éric Gagnon, Hélène Belleau, Aline Vézina. 2006. "Families' Values and Attitudes Regarding Responsibility for the Frail Elderly: Implications for Aging Policy." *Journal of Aging and Social Policy* 18(3/4): 59–78.

Harrington, Charlene. 2002. Unpublished analysis of 1997 deficiency statistics.

_____. 2001."Does Investor Ownership of Nursing Homes Compromise the Quality of Care?" *American Journal of Public Health* 91(9): 1453.

Havens, Betty. 2002. "Users of Long-Term Care." In Marion Stephenson and Eleanor Sawyer, eds., *Continuing the Care: The Issues and Challenges for Long-Term Care*. Ottawa, ON: CHA Press.

Health Canada. 2004. "What Is Continuing Care?" First Nations and Inuit Health, Health Canada. http://www.hc-sc.gc.ca/fnih-spni/pubs/home-domicile/2004_info_contin_care-soins/index_e.html.

Hillmer, Michael P., Walter P. Wodchis, Sudeep S. Gill, Geoffrey M. Anderson and Paula A. Rochon. 2005. "Nursing Home Profit Status and Quality of Care: Is There Any Evidence of an Association? *Medical Care Research and Review* 62: 2 (April): 139–66.

Hollander, Marcus. 2002. "The Continuum of Care: An Integrated System of Service Delivery." In Marion Stephenson and Eleanor Sawyer, eds., *Continuing the Care: The Issues and Challenges for Long-Term Care*. Ottawa, ON: CHA Press.

Huber, Manfred. 2005. "The Need to Improve the Comparability of Long-Term Care Expenditure Data: Recent Estimates from a Selection of OECD Countries and Follow-Up Work." Paris: Organization for Economic Cooperation and Development.

Jervis, Lori L., Yvonne M. Jackson and Spero M. Manson. 2002. "Need for, Availability of, and Barriers to the Provision of Long-Term Care for Older American Indians." *Journal of Cross Cultural Gerontology* 17(4): 295–311.

Keating N., J. Fast, D. Dosman and J. Eales. 2001. "Services Provided by Informal and Formal Caregivers to Seniors in Residential Continuing Care." *Canadian Journal on Aging* 20: 23–45.

Kelly, Len, and Judith Brown. 2002. "Listening to Native Patients: Changing in Physicians' Understanding and Behaviour." *Canadian Family Physician* 48: 1645–52.

Kite, S. 2006. "Palliative Care for Older People." *Age and Ageing* 35(5): 459–60.

Kittay, Eva Feder, with Bruce Jennings and Angela A. Wasunna. 2005. "Dependency, Difference and the Global Ethic of Longterm Care." *The Journal of Political Philosophy* 13(4): 443–69.

Kodner, Dennis. 2006. "Whole System Approaches to Health and Social Care Partnerships for the Frail Elderly: An Exploration of North American Models and Lessons." *Health and Social Care in the Community* 14(5): 384–90.

Kreig, B., D. Martz and L. McCallum. 2007. "Access to Health Services for Elderly Metis Women in Buffalo Narrows, Saskátchewan." Prairie Women's Centre of Excellence, Winnipeg.

Levin, Ron, and Margot Herbert. 2004. "The Experience of Urban Aboriginals with Health Care Services in Canada: Implications for Social Work Practice." *Social Work in Health Care* 39(1/2): 165–79.

Little, Margaret.1998. *No Car, No Radio, No Liquor Permit: The Moral Regulation of Single Mothers in Ontario, 1920–1997.* Toronto: Oxford University Press.

Lopez, Steven. 2006. "Emotional Labor and Organized Emotional Care: Conceptualizing Nursing Home Care Work." *Work and Occupations* 33(2): 133–60.

MacKinnon, Melanie. 2005. "A First Nations Voice in the Present Creates Healing in the Future." *Canadian Journal of Public Health* 96: S13–S16.

Magilvy, J.K., and J.A. Congdon. 2000. "The Crisis Nature of Health Care Transitions for Rural Older Adults." *Public Health Nursing* 17(5): 336–45.

Manitoba Health. 2007a. "Annual Statistics 2005-2006." Health Information Management, Manitoba Health. http://www.gov.mb.ca/health/annstats/200506/.

_____. 2007b. "Personal Care Services: A Guide to Services and Charges in Manitoba." Manitoba Health. http://www.gov.mb.ca/health/personalcare-services/.

_____. 2006. "Manitoba Launches New $98-Million Long-Term Care Strategy for Seniors: Aging in Place to Provide $80 million in Capital Construction, Expanded Community Programs, Over 1,110 More Spaces in Winnipeg." News Release, Manitoba Health. http://www.gov.mb.ca/chc/press/top/2006/01/2006-01-26-03.html.

McGrail, Kimberlyn, Margaret J. McGregor, Marcy Cohen, Robert Tate and Lisa A. Ronald. 2007. "For-profit versus Not-for-profit Delivery of Long-term Care." *Canadian Medical Association Journal* 176: 1(January 2): 57–58.

McGregor, Margaret J., Marcy Cohen, Kimberlyn McGrail, Anne Marie Broemeling, Reva N. Adler, Michael Schulzer, Lisa Ronald, Yuri Cvitkovich and Mary Beck. 2005. "Staffing Levels in Not-for-profit and For-profit Long-Term Care Facilities: Does Type of Ownership Matter?" *Canadian Medical Association Journal* 172 (5/March 1): 645–49.

McKay, Paul. 2003a. "Ontario's Nursing Home Crisis." *Ottawa Citizen*, April 26.

_____. 2003b. "Ontario's Nursing Home Crisis — Part 6." *Ottawa Citizen*, May 1.

Ministry of Health and Social Affairs, Sweden. 2007. *Care of the Elderly in Sweden.* Fact sheet. Government Offices of Sweden.

Ministry of Health, British Columbia. 2007a. "Community Care and Assisted Living Act." British Columbia Ministry of Health. http://www.health.gov.bc.ca/ccf/ccal/ccala.html.

_____. 2007b. "Home and Community Care Guide: A Guide to Your Care." British Columbia Ministry of Health Services. http://www.healthservices.gov.bc.ca/hcc/index.html.

_____. 2004. "A Profile of Seniors in BC." Victoria, BC: British Columbia Ministry of Health.

MOHLTC (Ministry of Health and Long-Term Care), Ontario. 2008. "Seniors' Care:

Home, Community and Residential Care Services for Seniors." Ministry of Health and Long-Term Care (MOHLTC). http://www.health.gov.on.ca/english/public/program/ltc/ltc_mn.html.

Moos, R., and S. Lemke. 1994. "Ownership, Size and Facility Quality." In R. Moos and S. Lemke, eds., *Group Residences for Older Adults: Physical Features, Policies and Social Climate.* New York: Oxford University Press.

Moss, S.Z., and M.S. Moss. 2007. "Being a Man in Long-Term Care." *Journal of Aging Studies* 21(1): 43–54.

Murphy, Janice M. 2006. *Residential Care Quality: A Review of the Literature on Nurse and Personal Care Staffing and Quality of Care.* Nursing Directorate, British Columbia Ministry of Health. November.

NAHO (National Aboriginal Health Organization). March 2002. "Moving Forward by Building Strengths: A Discussion Document on Aboriginal Hospice Palliative Care." Ottawa, Ontario.

National Coordinating Group on Health Care Reform and Women. 2002. *Women and Home Care: Why Does Home Care Matter to Women?* http://www.womenandhealthcarereform.ca/publications/why-hc-matter.pdf.

_____. 2000. *Women and Health Care Reform.* http://www.womenandhealthcarereform.ca/publications/women-hcren.pdf.

NBHW (National Board of Health and Welfare). 2008. *Mot en mer jämställd sjukvård och socialtjänst,* [Towards More Gender Equality in Health Care and Social Services.] Stockholm: National Board of Health and Welfare.

_____. 2007a. *Äldre — vård och omsorg 2006. Statstik.* [Care and Services for Elderly People. Statistics.] Stockholm: National Board for Health and Welfare.

_____. 2007b. *Verksamhetens kvalitet.* [Open Comparisons of Care for Older People. Quality of the Services.] Stockholm: National Board for Health and Welfare.

_____. 2007c. *Äldres deltagande i matlagningen på gruppboenden* [Elderly Persons' Participation in Cooking in Group Dwellings.] Stockholm: National Board for Health and Welfare.

_____. 2007d. *Current Developments in Care of the Elderly in Sweden.* Stockholm: National Board of Health and Welfare.

OECD (Organization for Economic Cooperation and Development). 2005. *Long Term Care for Older People.* Paris: OECD.

OHC (Ontario Health Coalition). 2008. *Violence, Insufficient Care, and Downloading of Heavy Care Patients: An Evaluation of Increasing Need and Inadequate Standards in Ontario's Nursing Homes.* Toronto, ON: Ontario Health Coalition

_____. 2007. "Backgrounder on Long Term Care Facilities Minimum Care Standards." September 9. www.ontariohealthcoalition.ca.

_____. 2002. "Ownership Matters: Lessons from Ontario's Long-Term Care Facilities." Ontario Health Coalition (OHC).

Ontario Ministry of Health and Long-Term Care. 2007. "McGuinty Government Eliminating Multi-bed Wards Through Upgrades at Older Long-Term Care Homes Across Province." July 31. http://www.health.gov.on.ca/english/media/news_releases/archives/nr_07/jul/nr_20070731.html.

_____. 2004. *Commitment to Care: A Plan for Long-Term Care in Ontario.* Prepared by Monique Smith, Parliamentary Assistant.

Ontario Non-Profit Housing Association (ONPHA). 2007. *Sound the Alarm Bells: Critical*

*Need for Recruitment and Succession in the Ontario Non-Profit Housing Sector.* August. http://www.onpha.on.ca/issues_position_papers/housing.

Parsons, Talcott. 1951. *The Social System.* London: Routledge and Kegan Paul.

Pitters, Sandra. 2002. "Long-Term Care Facilities." In Marion Stephenson and Eleanor Sawyer, eds., *Continuing the Care: The Issues and Challenges for Long-Term Care.* Ottawa, ON: CHA Press.

Premier's Council on Aging and Seniors' Issues. 2006. *Aging Well in British Columbia.* British Columbia. November.

Prince, Holly, and Mary Lou Kelley. 2006. "Palliative Care in First Nations Communities: The Perspectives and Experiences of Aboriginal Elders and the Educational Needs of Their Community Caregivers." Lakehead University.

Prokop, Shelley Thomas, Erika Haug, Michelle Hogan, Jason McCarthy and Lorraine McDonald. 2004. "Aboriginal Women and Home Care." In Karen Grant et al., eds., *Caring For/Caring About: Women, Home Care and Unpaid Caregiving.* Aurora, ON: Garamond.

PWC (PricewaterhouseCoopers). 2001. "Report of a Study to Review Levels of Service and Responses to Need in a Sample of Ontario Long-Term Care Facilities and Selected Comparators." PricewaterhouseCoopers, LLP.

RAMQ. 2008. "Financial Contribution - Accommodated Adults."http://www.ramq. gouv.qc.ca/en/citoyens/contributionetaidefinancieres/index.shtml.

_____. 2007. "Financial Contribution — Accommodated Adults." http://www. ramq.gouv.qc.ca/en/impression.htm.

RHS (Regional Longitudinal Health Survey). 2002–2003. *First Nations Seniors Health and Well-being.* http://www.rhs-ers.ca/english/pdf/rhs2002-03reports/rhs2002-03-technicalreport-afn.pdf.

Robinson, Julie, and Karl Pillemer. 2007. "Job Satisfaction and Intention to Quit Among Nursing Home Staff: Do Special Care Units Make a Difference?" *The Journal of Applied Gerontology* 26(February 1): 95–112.

Romanow, Roy J., Q.C. 2002. *Building Values: The Future of Health Care in Canada.* Final Report. Commission on the Future of Health Care in Canada. November. http://www.cbc.ca/healthcare/final_report.pdf.

Roos, N.P., L. Stranc, S. Peterson, L. Mitchell, B. Bogdanovic and E. Shapiro. 2001. "A Look at Home Care in Manitoba." Winnipeg: Manitoba Centre for Health Policy and Evaluation.

Roscelli, Margaret. 2005. "Political Advocacy and Research Both Needed to Address Provincial Gaps in Service: Manitoba First Nations Personal Care Homes." *Canadian Journal of Public Health* 96 (Supplement 1): S55–S59.

SALAR (Swedish Association of Local Authorities and Regions). 2007. *Care of the Elderly in Sweden Today.* Stockholm: Swedish Association of Local Authorities and Regions.

Sawyer, Eleanor, and Marion Stephenson. 1995, rev. ed. 2002. *Continuing the Care: The Issues and Challenges for Long-Term Care.* Ottawa: Canadian Nurses Association.

Shannon, David W. 2007. *Six Degrees of Dignity: Disability in an Age of Freedom.* Ottawa: Creative Bound International.

Shapiro, E. and R.B. Tate. 1995. "Monitoring the Outcomes of Quality in Nursing Homes Using Administrative Data." *Canadian Journal on Aging* 14: 755–68.

Sharkey, S. 2008. *People Caring for People: Impacting the Quality of Life and Care of Residents of Long-Term Care Homes. A Report of the Independent Review of Staffing and Care Standards for Long-Term Care Homes in Ontario.* Toronto, ON: Ministry of Health and Long-term Care.

Sikorska-Simmons, Elzbieta. 2006a. "The Effects of Organizational Context on Autonomy-Enhancing Policies in Assisted Living." *Journal of Aging Studies* 20: 217–226.

_____. 2006b. "Linking Resident Satisfaction to Staff Perceptions of the Work Environment in Assisted Living: A Multilevel Analysis." *The Gerontologist* 46(5): 590–98.

Smith, Monique. 2004. "Commitment to Care: A Plan for Long-Term Care in Ontario." Toronto: Ministry of Health and Long-Term Care.

Smye, V., and W. Mussell. 2001. "Aboriginal Mental Health: What Works Best — A Discussion Paper." The Aboriginal Mental Health Best Practices Working Group, Mheccu, Funded by Adult Mental Health Division, Ministry of Health, Victoria, B.C.

Smyer, Tish, and Thomas E. Stenvig. 2007. "Health Care for American Indian Elders: An Overview of Cultural Influences and Policy Issues." *Home Health Care Management and Practice* 20(1): 27–33.

Smylie, Janet. 2001. "A Guide for Health Professionals Working with Aboriginal Peoples, SOGC Policy Statement Executive Summary: The Sociocultural Context of Aboriginal Peoples in Canada." *Journal of Obstetrics and Gynecology Canada* (January): 1–15.

Smylie, Janet, and Marcia Anderson. 2006. "Understanding the Health of Indigenous Peoples in Canada: Key Methodological and Conceptual Challenges." *Canadian Medical Association Journal* 175(6): 602–605.

Somerville, N. 2007. "Changes in Long-term Care 'Scary' for Seniors; Vital Medical and Personal Services Being Deinsured and Privatized as Province Moves from Nursing Homes to 'Aging-in-Place' Care," *Edmonton Journal,* June 6: A17.

Statistics Canada. 2007a. "A Portrait of Seniors." *The Daily Tuesday.* February 27: 1–4.

_____. 2007b. *Aboriginal Peoples. Seniors: Foundations of Their Communities.* October 7. http://www41.statcan.ca/2007/10000/ceb10000_002_e.htm.

_____. 2007c. *Residential Care Facilities 2005/2006.*

_____. 2006. *A Portrait of Seniors in Canada.* http://www.statcan.ca/bsolc/english/ bsolc?catno=89-519-X.

_____. 2003. *Aboriginal Peoples Survey 2001 — Initial Findings: Well-being of the Nonreserve Aboriginal Population.* http://www.statcan.ca/english/freepub/89-589-XIE/ index.htm.

_____. 2001. *Census Aboriginal Population Profile.* http://www12.statcan.ca/english/ profil01ab/PlaceSearchForm1.cfm.

Swedish Social Insurance Agency. 2008. *Bostadstillägg till pensionärer.* [Housing Supplements for Pensioners.] Fact sheet, updated March 3.

Szebehely, Marta. 2005a. "Care as Employment and Welfare Provision: Child Care and Elder Care in Sweden at the Dawn of the 21st Century." In Hanne Dahl, Marlene and Tine Rask Eriksen, eds., *Dilemmas of Care in the Nordic Welfare State.* Aldershot: Ashgate.

_____. 2005b. "Anhörigas betalda och obetalda äldreomsorgsinsatser" [Unpaid and

Paid Family Care for Elderly People.] In *Forskarrapporter till Jämställdhetspolitiska utredningen* [Research Reports for the Inquiry on Gender Equality Policy.] Government Report SOU 2005: 66. Stockholm: Fritzes.

Tellis-Nayak, V. 2007. "A Person-Centered Workplace: The Foundation for Person-Centered Caregiving in Long-Term Care." *Journal of American Medical Directors Association* 8(1): 46–54.

Tesh, Syliva. 1988. *Hidden Arguments: Political Ideology and Disease Prevention Policy*. London: Rutgers University Press.

*Toronto Star*. 2008. "Nursing Home Crackdown." May 16: A1.

Trocmé, Nico, Della Knoke and Cindy Blackstock. 2004. "Pathways to the Overrepresentation of Aboriginal Children in Canada's Child Welfare System." *Social Service Review* (December): 577–600.

Trydegård, G-B. 2003. "Swedish Care Reforms in the 1990s. A First Evaluation of their Consequences for Elderly People." *Revue Française des Affaires Sociales* 4: 443–60.

Tyler, Denise, Victoria Parker, Ryann Engle, Gary Brandeis, Elaine Hickey, Amy Rosen, Fei Wang and Dan Berlowitz. 2006. "An Exploration of Job Design in Long-Term Care Facilities and its Effects on Nursing Satisfaction." *Health Care Management Review* 31(2): 137–44.

VAC (Veterans Affairs Canada). 2002. "VAC's Approach to Long-Term Care." In *Salute!* Veterans Affairs Canada (VAC).http://www.vac-acc.gc.ca/clients/sub. cfm?source=salute/summer2002/long_term_care.

_____. 1997. "Client Profile of Veterans Residing in Long-term Care Facilities." Veterans Affairs Canada. http://www.vac-acc.gc.ca/providers/sub. cfm?source=needs/ltc&CFID=18569942&CFTOKEN=62231997.

Vladeck, Bruce. 2004. "Foreword." In Thomas Edward Gass, *Nobody's Home: Candid Reflections of a Nursing Home Aide*. Ithaca: Cornell University Press.

_____. 2003. "Unloving Care Revisited: The Persistence of Culture." In Audrey S. Weiner and Judah L. Ronch, eds., *Culture Change in Long-Term Care*. New York: Haworth Press.

Vogal, Donna. 1999. "Unfulfilled Promise: How Health Care Reforms of the 1990s are Failing Community and Continuing Care in BC." In *Without Foundation* (Vancouver: Canadian Centre for Policy Alternatives), 39.

Vosko, Leah, ed. 2006. *Precarious Employment: Understanding Labour Market Insecurity in Canada*. Montreal: McGill-Queens University Press.

WHO (World Health Organization). 2004. *Better Palliative Care for Older People*. http://www.euro.who.int/document/E82933.pdf.

WRHA (Winnipeg Regional Health Authority). 2007. "Personal Care Home Program." Winnipeg Regional Health Authority. http://www.wrha.mb.ca/ltc/pch/index. php.

YHSS (Yukon Health and Social Services). 2007. "Residential Care Services." Yukon Health and Social Services. http://www.hss.gov.yk.ca/programs/continuing/ residential/.